THE AMERICAN ACADEMY OF ORTHOPAEDIC SURGEONS

Instructional
Course
Lectures

Volume XXIX   1980

THE AMERICAN ACADEMY OF ORTHOPAEDIC SURGEONS

Instructional Course Lectures

Volume XXIX   1980

With 287 illustrations

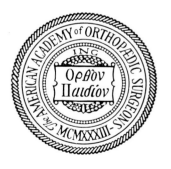

The C. V. Mosby Company

ST. LOUIS · TORONTO · LONDON   1980

Contributors

Charles R. Clark, M.D.

Department of Orthopaedic Surgery, University of Iowa Hospitals and Clinics, Iowa City, Iowa

Stephen F. Gunther, M.D.

Associate Professor of Orthopaedic Surgery, The George Washington University School of Medicine; Chairman, Department of Orthopaedic Surgery, Washington Hospital Center, Washington, D.C.

Kevin D. Harrington, M.D.

Clinical Assistant Professor of Orthopaedic Surgery, University of California, San Francisco, California

Leslie J. Harris, M.D.

Assistant Professor, Department of Orthopaedics, University of Southern California School of Medicine, Los Angeles, California

Hill Hastings, II, M.D.

Hand Surgery Service, Department of Orthopaedic Surgery, Massachusetts General Hospital; Clinical Fellow in Orthopaedic Surgery, Harvard Medical School, Boston, Massachusetts

Gordon A. Hunter, M.B., F.R.C.S., F.R.C.S.(C)

Associate Professor of Surgery, University of Toronto; Orthopaedic Division, Sunnybrook Medical Centre, Toronto, Ontario, Canada

John D. Loeser, M.D.

Associate Professor, Department of Neurological Surgery, University of Washington, Seattle, Washington

G. Dean MacEwen, M.D.

Medical Director, Alfred I. duPont Institute of The Nemours Foundation, Wilmington, Delaware; Clinical Professor of Orthopaedic Surgery, Thomas Jefferson University, Philadelphia, Pennsylvania

Marvin H. Meyers, M.D.

Professor of the Division of Orthopaedic Surgery, The University of Texas Health Science Center at Dallas, Southwestern Medical School, Dallas, Texas

Raymond T. Morrissy, M.D.

Associate Professor, Department of Orthopaedic Surgery and Pediatrics, University of Arkansas for Medical Sciences, Little Rock, Arkansas

Terence M. Murphy, M.B., Ch.B., F.F.A.R.C.S.

Associate Professor of Anesthesiology, Acting Director of Pain Clinic, University of Washington, Seattle, Washington

Carl L. Nelson, M.D.

Professor and Chairman, Department of Orthopaedic Surgery, University of Arkansas for Medical Sciences, Little Rock, Arkansas

Robert J. Neviaser, M.D.

Professor of Orthopaedic Surgery, Director of Hand and Upper Extremity Service, The George Washington University Medical Center, Washington, D.C.

John A. Ogden, M.D.

Section of Orthopaedics, Skeletal Growth and Development Study Unit, Yale University School of Medicine, New Haven, Connecticut

Joseph Schatzker, M.D., B.Sc.(Med.), F.R.C.S.(C)

Associate Professor of Surgery, University of Toronto; Active Staff, Division of Orthopaedic Surgery, The Wellesley Hospital, Toronto, Ontario, Canada

Robert S. Siffert, M.D.

Professor and Chairman, Department of Orthopaedics, Mount Sinai School of Medicine, The City University of New York, New York, New York

Franklin H. Sim, M.D.

Consultant, Department of Orthopedics, Mayo Clinic and Mayo Foundation; Associate Professor of Orthopedic Surgery, Mayo Medical School, Rochester, Minnesota

Richard J. Smith, M.D.

Clinical Professor, Orthopaedic Surgery, Harvard Medical School; Chief of Hand Surgery Service, Department of Orthopaedic Surgery, Massachusetts General Hospital, Boston, Massachusetts

Wayne O. Southwick, M.D.

Section of Orthopaedic Surgery, Skeletal Growth and Development Study Unit, Yale University School of Medicine, New Haven, Connecticut

Dan M. Spengler, M.D.

Associate Professor, Department of Orthopaedics, University of Washington School of Medicine, Seattle, Washington

Richard N. Stauffer, M.D.

Consultant, Department of Orthopedics, Mayo Clinic and Mayo Foundation; Associate Professor of Orthopedic Surgery, Mayo Medical School, Rochester, Minnesota

Dana M. Street, M.D.

Professor of Orthopedic Surgery and Rehabilitation, Loma Linda University; Chief, Orthopedic Section, Jerry L. Pettis Memorial Veterans Hospital, Loma Linda, California

Marvin Tile, M.D., B.Sc.(Med.), F.R.C.S.(C)

Chief Orthopaedic Surgeon, Sunnybrook Medical Centre; Associate Professor of Surgery, University of Toronto, Toronto, Ontario, Canada

Preface

The annual Instructional Course Program of the Academy is a major and outstanding continuing medical education activity. From it, presentations are selected for publication in this volume by the Instructional Course Committee. Obviously, the text does not include all of the courses presented in any one year. A number of courses do not lend themselves to publication; to include some others would create a duplication of previously published material.

The Committee selects subjects with an emphasis on overall interest to those in the practice of orthopaedic surgery. In addition, an author's ability to convey information in a concise manner to the reader is a factor in the selection process. Further emphasis is placed on proven methods rather than on innovations that have not had the test of time or experience. Historically, this publication has not been a sounding board for unproven techniques or theories.

In addition to any benefits a reader may receive from information in a book of this type, time has shown the *Instructional Course Lectures* series serves as a good source of pertinent references to many subjects related to the musculoskeletal system. Readers with a desire to pursue subjects in greater depth will find this resource helpful.

The material presented in this publication has been made available by the American Academy of Orthopaedic Surgeons for educational purposes only. This material is not intended to represent the only, or necessarily the best, methods or procedures appropriate for the medical situations discussed; rather it is intended to present an approach, view, statement, or opinion of the authors that may be helpful to others who face similar situations.

We are especially grateful to all authors, without whom the *Instructional Course Lectures* series would not be possible.

Committee on Instructional Courses
Hanes H. Brindley, *Editor*
David G. Murray, *Chairman*
Joseph A. Kopta
Victor H. Frankel
C. McCollister Evarts

Contents

THE AMERICAN ACADEMY OF ORTHOPAEDIC SURGEONS

Instructional
Course
Lectures

Volume XXIX   1980

Chapter 1

Fractures of the neck of the femur

Part I

Displaced fractures of the femoral neck—internal fixation or hemiarthroplasty?

GORDON A. HUNTER

THE ROLE OF INTERNAL FIXATION AND PROSTHETIC REPLACEMENT

The displaced fracture of the femoral neck still presents problems to the orthopaedic surgeon and is of significance both economically to health service facilities and socially to patients and their relatives.

Nonoperative treatment should be restricted to those patients with severe mental illness or retardation, those living a bed-chair existence, or in the rare situation when deep pressure sores prevent a safe surgical incision.[27]

Operative treatment improves the comfort of the patient by relief of pain and facilitates nursing care, thus reducing the length of stay in an expensive "active treatment" hospital bed. It is debatable whether it reduces the incidence of thromboembolism, which may be in excess of 50% after surgical treatment of femoral neck fractures.[24]

Operative treatment should be carried out as soon as practical after assessment by either the internist or anesthetist. Early treatment should relieve the patient's discomfort and reduces further damage to the blood supply of the femoral head.

The possibilities of surgical treatment include the following:

1. Closed reduction and internal fixation
2. Open reduction and internal fixation, with or without a muscle pedicle graft supplemented by iliac bone chips[21]
3. Hemiarthroplasty, with or without the use of cement
4. Single assembly hip replacement of the Bateman or Giliberty type, with or without cement
5. Total hip replacement

Closed reduction of the fracture

Garden[12] stated that "achievement of accurate reduction was largely a matter of chance." Flynn[10] recommended the following method:

1. Gentle flexion of the limb to beyond 90 degrees of flexion with 10 degrees abduction and neutral rotation.
2. Traction in the line of the neck of the femur.
3. Gentle internal rotation as the leg is extended. Then the leg should be fixed in extension, internal rotation, and 10 degrees of abduction.

This method is less traumatic than that described by Leadbetter.[17] The reduction should then be checked by image intensifier if possible. Concerning the acceptability of reduction, Garden[13] has now come to rely on the appearance of the fragments as seen in a lateral radiograph as the best guide to the prognosis of union of the fracture.

I prefer to place a guide wire in the middle of the head and neck in both planes. It should be remembered that the head of the femur normally shows a slight posteroinferior overhang on the neck.[12] I prefer to use a sliding screw-type device and fix the plate to the shaft of the femur with two or three screws, often combined with a threaded pin to stabilize the fracture (Fig. 1-1).

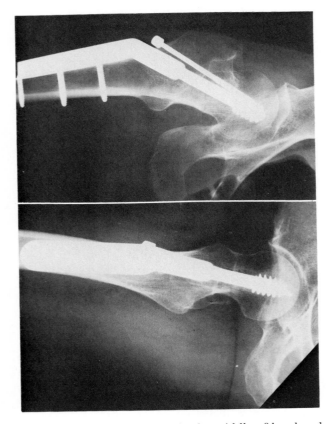

Fig. 1-1. Placement of screw in the middle of head and neck in both planes. If the screw appears to be low in the head and neck, it may be combined with a threaded pin to stabilize the fracture.

The screw should be inserted just below the articular surface of the femoral head.

I use prophylactic antibiotics for 2 or 3 days and anticoagulants in selected high-risk patients.

I allow early weight bearing as soon as practical and transfer the patient to a convalescent hospital 2 to 3 weeks after the operation.

COMPLICATIONS OF INTERNAL FIXATION

Avascular necrosis, with or without late segmental collapse. Published figures of rate of incidence report a range of 6% to 84%,[8,26] averaging approximately 25% to 30%. It should be remembered that avascular necrosis may be partial or complete. It is frequently asymptomatic, and, even if symptomatic, it does not always require reconstructive surgery.

Nonunion. The reported incidence varies from 5% to 35%,[20,21] but if these figures are reversed, union may occur in 65% to 95% of patients. From

Table 1. Comparative deep infection rate in reported series of fractures of the neck of the femur treated by prosthetic replacement and internal fixation

	Primary prosthesis	*Internal fixation*
Hunter[14]	9%	0%
Raine[23]	6%	0%
Arnold et al.[2]	8% (approximately)	0.5%
Fielding et al.[9]	8%	0%
Hunter[15]	9%	3%

Table 2. Incidence of dislocation of hemiarthroplasty

Lunt[18]	10%
Wrighton and Woodyard[32]	3%
Raine[23]	8%
Hunter[15]	7%
Chan and Hoskinson[5]	8%
D'Arcy and Devas[7]	2%
Bracey[4]	7%
Hunter[16]	11%

a large review of 1503 patients,[3] 67% of Type III and IV fractures united, often demonstrating delayed union. Surprisingly enough, a delay of up to 1 week before operation had no significant effect on the incidence of nonunion.

Infection. The reported incidence varies from 0% to 3%.[14,15] Malcolm and Schatzker[19] have recently stressed that subluxation or dislocation of the femoral head after internal fixation of the fracture is an important clue to the diagnosis of deep infection.

Hemiarthroplasty

If the complications of closed reduction and internal fixation are so frequent, why should we not advise routine excision of the femoral head and replacement with a femoral prosthesis?

COMPLICATIONS

The reasons we should not adopt this method of treatment routinely relate to the problems arising from deep infection, dislocation of the prosthesis, problems of revision, especially with cemented prostheses, and mortality figures.

Infection. The incidence of deep infection after prosthetic replacement has been reported to be as high as 42%[22] and compares most unfavorably with the rate of incidence after closed reduction and internal fixation (Table 1).

Table 3. Comparative mortality figures after internal fixation, primary and secondary replacement

Author	Time period	Internal fixation	Primary prosthesis	Secondary prosthesis
Garcia et al.[11]	6 Months	4%	18%	
Stein and Costen[30]	Postoperative		12%	1%
Hunter[14]	6 Months	15%	41%	10%
Raine[23]	6 Months	12%	33%	
Arnold et al.[2]	In Hospital	1%	11%	0.4%
Hunter[15]	6 Months	15%	24%	10%
Albright and Weinstein[1]	1 Year		41%	10%
Bracey[4]	6 Months	21%	30%	5%

Dislocation of the prosthesis. The reported incidence in recent literature varies from 2% to 11%[7,16] (Table 2). When dislocation is associated with sepsis, the outcome is invariably fatal.

In view of the high incidence of dislocation reported by Whittaker et al.[31] and Coughlin and Templeton,[6] I would avoid prosthetic replacement in patients with Parkinson's disease.

Problems of revision after prosthetic replacement. Unlike the revision procedure after failed internal fixation, in which a number of alternatives are available, a failed hemiarthroplasty must be converted to a total hip replacement, provided that sepsis is excluded as a possible cause of pain. Smith and Amstutz[29] reviewed 41 failed femoral hemiarthroplasties converted to total hip replacements. They reported intraoperative femoral shaft fractures, two dislocations, and one deep infection. There was a high incidence of loosening of the femoral component, and technically imperfect cement fixation was recorded in 30 of 41 hips in the first postoperative radiograph.

Mortality rate. The mortality rate 6 months after primary prosthetic replacement ranges from 18% to 41%.[11,14] These figures should be compared to the lower mortality figures at the same time period after internal fixation and after secondary prosthetic replacement (Table 3).

Other complications. An analysis of the incidence and problems of loosening of the femoral prosthesis, acetabular erosion, and fractures of the femoral shaft around the prosthesis during or after the operation will not be presented here.

USE OF CEMENT

Whether or not to routinely cement a prosthesis has been well discussed by Sledge,[28] but it is interesting that in a recent personal review,[16] there was little difference in the results and complications of 55 patients with uncemented Moore prostheses and 45 patients with cemented Thompson prostheses for displaced femoral neck fractures.

CONCLUSIONS

I would remind you that Senn[25] pointed out that "the only cause for nonunion of intracapsular fractures is our inability to maintain perfect coaptation and immobilization of the fragments until bony union has taken place". Almost all displaced femoral neck fractures should be treated by careful closed reduction and internal fixation whenever possible. Accurate reduction of the fracture is more important than the actual instruments used for internal fixation, which may depend on the personal preference of the individual surgeon.

In the management of the patient with a fresh displaced fracture of the femoral neck, I would consider alternative procedures only in the following circumstances:

1. Failure of closed reduction
2. Delay of more than a few days after the accident, to avoid problems of avascular necrosis and nonunion
3. Pathologic fracture due to metastatic disease
4. A "high-level" subcapital fracture
5. A fracture of the neck of the femur associated with dislocation of the femoral head
6. Pre-existing Paget's disease or arthritis associated with a fracture of the neck of the femur

I would remind you that the only conditions preventing further procedures on the hip joint after fracture of the neck of the femur are a dead patient and an infected hip joint. We should, therefore, strive to reduce the incidence of infection, morbidity, and mortality in this common but serious fracture. The best way of doing this at the present time is to reduce the fracture accurately as soon as possible and to treat the fracture by internal fixation.

REFERENCES

1. Albright, J. P., and Weinstein, S. L.: Treatment for fixation complications. Femoral neck fractures, Arch. Surg. **110:**30, 1975.
2. Arnold, W. D., Lyden, J. P., and Minkoff, J.: Treatment of intracapsular fractures of the femoral neck, J. Bone Joint Surg. **56-A:**254, 1974.
3. Barnes, R., Brown, J. T., Garden, R. S., and Nicoll, E. A.: Subcapital fracture of the femur, J. Bone Joint Surg. **58-B:**2, 1976.
4. Bracey, D. J.: A comparison of internal fixation and prosthetic replacement in the treatment of displaced subcapital fractures, Injury **9:**1, 1977.
5. Chan, R. N. W., and Hoskinson, J.: Thompson prosthesis for fractured neck of femur, J. Bone Joint Surg. **57-B:**437, 1975.
6. Coughlin, L. P., and Templeton, J.: Hip fractures in patient with Parkinson's disease. Paper presented to the Canadian Orthopaedic Association Meeting, Toronto, 1977.
7. D'Arcy, J., and Devas, M.: Treatment of fractures of the femoral neck by replacement with the Thompson prosthesis, J. Bone Joint Surg. **58-B:**279, 1977.
8. Deyerle, W. M.: Plate and peripheral pins in hip fractures: two plane reduction, total impaction, and absolute fixation. In Adams, J. P., editor: Current practice in orthopaedic surgery, vol. III, St. Louis, 1966, The C. V. Mosby Co., pp. 173-207.
9. Fielding, J. W., Wilson, S. A., and Ratzan, S.: A continuing end-result study of displaced intracapsular fractures of the neck of the femur treated with the Pugh nail, J. Bone Joint Surg. **56-A:**1464, 1974.
10. Flynn, M.: A new method of reduction of fractures of the neck of the femur based on anatomical studies of the hip joint, Injury **5:**309, 1974.
11. Garcia, A., Jr., Neer, C. S., and Ambrose, G. B.: Displaced intracapsular fractures of the neck of the femur. Part I. Mortality and morbidity, J. Trauma **1:**28, 1961.
12. Garden, R. S.: Malreduction and avascular necrosis in subcapital fractures of the femur, J. Bone Joint Surg. **53-B:**183, 1971.
13. Garden, R. S.: Selective surgery in medial fractures of the femoral neck. A review, Injury **9:**5, 1977.
14. Hunter, G. A.: A comparison of the use of internal fixation and prosthetic replacement for fresh fractures of the neck of the femur, Br. J. Surg. **56:**229, 1969.
15. Hunter, G. A.: A further comparison of the use of internal fixation and prosthetic replacement for fresh fractures of the neck of the femur, Br. J. Surg. **61:**382, 1974.
16. Hunter, G. A.: Should we abandon primary prosthetic replacement for fresh displaced fractures of the neck of the femur? (In press.)
17. Leadbetter, G. W.: A treatment for fracture of the neck of the femur, J. Bone Joint Surg. **15:**931, 1933.
18. Lunt, H. R. W.: The use of prosthetic replacement of the head of the femur as primary treatment for subcapital fractures, Injury **3:**107, 1978.
19. Malcolm, B. W., and Schatzker, J.: Subluxation and dislocation of the hip. A complication following hip pinning. Paper presented to the Canadian Orthopaedic Association Meeting, Vancouver, 1978.
20. Metz, C. W., Sellers, T. D., Feagin, J. A., Levine, M. I., Onkey, R. G., Dwyer, J. W., and Eberhard, E. J.: The displaced intracapsular fracture of the neck of the femur. Experience with the Deyerle method of fixation in 63 cases, J. Bone Joint Surg. **52-A:**113, 1970.
21. Meyers, M. H., Harvey, J. P., Jr., and Moore, T. M.: Treatment of displaced subcapital and transcervical fractures of the femoral neck by muscle-pedicle-bone graft and internal fixation, J. Bone Joint Surg. **55-A:**257, 1973.
22. Niemann, K. M. W., and Mankin, H. J.: Fractures about the hip in an institutionalized patient population, J. Bone Joint Surg. **50-A:**1327, 1968.
23. Raine, G. E. T.: A comparison of internal fixation and prosthetic replacement for recent displaced subcapital fractures of the neck of the femur, Injury **5:**25, 1973.
24. Salzman, E. W., and Harris, W. H.: Prevention of thromboembolism in orthopaedic patients, J. Bone Joint Surg. **58-A:**903, 1976.
25. Senn, N.: Fractures of the neck of the femur with special reference to bony union after intracapsular fracture, Trans. Am. Surg. Assoc. **1:**333, 1883.
26. Sevitt, S.: Avascular necrosis and revascularization of the femoral head after intracapsular fractures, J. Bone Joint Surg. **46-B:**270, 1964.
27. Sherk, H. H., Crouse, F. R., and Probst, C.: The treatment of hip fractures in institutionalized patients, Orthop. Clin. North Am. **5:**543, 1974.
28. Sledge, C. B.: Discussion. In The Hip Society: The hip, vol. 5, St. Louis, 1977, The C. V. Mosby Co., pp. 124-126.
29. Smith, R. K., and Amstutz, H. C.: Total hip replacement following failed femoral hemiarthroplasty, Orthop. Transactions **2:**251, 1978.
30. Stein, A. H., Jr., and Costen, W. S.: Hip arthroplasty with the metallic prosthesis, J. Bone Joint Surg. **44-A:**1155, 1962.
31. Whittaker, R. P., Abeshaus, M. M., Scholl, H. W., and Chung, S. M. K.: Fifteen years experience with metallic endoprosthetic replacement of the femoral head for femoral neck fractures, J. Trauma **12:**799, 1972.
32. Wrighton, J. D., and Woodyard, J. E.: Prosthetic replacement for subcapital fractures of the femur. A comparative survey, Injury **2:**287, 1971.

Part II

Treatment by muscle pedicle graft and internal fixation

MARVIN H. MEYERS

Because of the continued high incidence of avascular necrosis and nonunion after open reduction and internal fixation of displaced femoral neck fractures, a literature review and study of this fracture was started in 1965. In spite of the endless introduction of innovative metallic fixatives, it was apparent that little headway had been made in reducing the incidence of these two undesirable complications. The rate of nonunion, 15% to 35%, and the rate of large segmental collapse, 30% of the cases that united, remained unchanged.

Most authors concluded that nonunion was caused by failure to maintain coaptation and immobilization of the fracture fragments prior to union. Other contributing factors that were suggested included the patient, type of fracture, technical errors in fixation, the healing mechanism, time from fracture to fixation, and premature weight bearing.

Authors were in agreement that accurate reduction, impaction of the fracture fragments af-

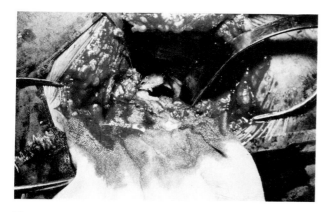

Fig. 1-2. Posterior neck defect with large cavity left after crushing of trabeculae in neck and head of femur.

ter reduction, and rigid fixation were essential if the best rate of union was to be obtained.

However, achievement of these goals is not always possible due to marked comminution of the posterior neck of the femur. This was identified in 70% of a series of fractures I treated by a muscle pedicle graft and internal fixation. Frequently, a large gap was noted in the posterior neck, which was devoid of bone (Fig. 1-2). This can be confirmed preoperatively on x-ray examination with good across-table lateral x-rays films of the involved hip. Anatomic reduction is not possible in the presence of severe posterior neck comminution, and impaction is only possible in two thirds or less of the opposing cortical rims at the fracture site. Although rigid fixation is desirable, the paucity and attenuation of the intramedullary trabeculae in the head fragment of the elderly patient makes this difficult to achieve. (Fig. 1-3).

A major obstacle to the solution of the "unsolved" fracture is the extent of damage to the blood supply of the head fragment following fracture. Many authors including Catto,[2] Calandruccio,[1] and Sevitt[9] have reported that two thirds of the heads, following fracture of the neck of the femur with displacement, are totally or subtotally avascular. More than one third are completely avascular. Thus, avascular necrosis of bone must occur within a few hours of injury. Union of the fracture and revascularization follow in most avascular femoral heads that are reduced and ad-

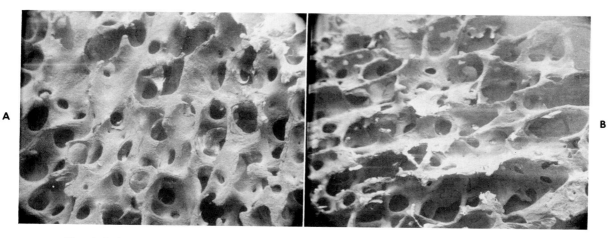

Fig. 1-3. Scanning electron microscopy section of macerated femoral heads (×20). **A,** Twenty-nine-year-old woman with average normal thickness and concentration of trabeculae. **B,** Sixty-eight-year-old woman with attenuation and decreased number of trabeculae.

equately fixed internally. Late segmental collapse of the femoral head, the troublesome complication of avascular necrosis, occurs at about 9 to 24 months after the injury in most cases.

This concept should be clearly understood. Avascular necrosis occurs within the first few hours after injury. Revascularization from the vascular distal fragment is a slow "creeping" process that cannot begin until the fracture is reduced and immobilized by metal fixation. Since revascularization of bone is a steady, orderly process dependent upon the ingrowth of capillaries along the framework of the intramedullary trabecular system, the defect subsequent to the comminution of the posterior neck must act as a barrier to the revascularization process in the proximal fragment. (See Fig. 1-2.) Thus, it can be hypothesized that nonunion in some cases and slow revascularization in others are due to the lack of bone in the large gap posteriorly.

In 1967, I was introduced to the muscle pedicle graft of the quadratus femoris muscle[3] as a means of providing an additional source of blood to the head fragment after femoral neck fracture when the blood supply was diminished or totally absent. This procedure permits the addition of supplemental iliac bone to fill the defect in the posterior neck, thereby providing a source of chemicals for new bone deposition and a scaffold for the ingrowth of capillaries in the revascularization process. The pedicle graft aids fracture stability by providing additional fixation.

Although it is well-established that avascular necrosis occurs immediately after the occurence of the fracture, the reason for late segmental collapse, which is rarely seen prior to 9 months after injury, is yet unknown. It is inappropriate at this point to engage in a long hypothetic discussion on the cause of late segmental collapse.

INDICATIONS FOR MUSCLE PEDICLE GRAFT

The indications for a muscle pedicle graft are (1) displaced fractures of the neck of the femur after closure of the proximal femoral epiphysis and (2) nondisplaced or impacted femoral neck fractures, when absence of a blood supply or severely impaired blood supply to the head fragment can be demonstrated. Technetium 99m sulfur colloid (SC) scans of the pelvis are 95% accurate in revealing the absence or severe damage of circulation in the femoral head[7] (Fig. 1-4).

CONTRAINDICATIONS FOR MUSCLE PEDICLE GRAFT

The muscle pedicle graft procedure is contraindicated in the following patients:
1. Nonwalkers or minimal walkers
2. Those with a short life expectancy
3. Those unable to cooperate in a postoperative rehabilitation program due to the following:
   a. Senility
   b. Psychosis
   c. Mental retardation
   d. Parkinsonism
   e. Cerebrovascular accident (CVA) with residual hemiplegia or spasticity
   f. Severe debility
4. Those with rheumatoid arthritis with severe joint involvement, pathologic fractures, or advanced degenerative osteoarthritis of the hip

ADVANTAGES

The muscle pedicle graft procedure has several advantages. It allows direct visualization of the posterior neck of the femur. Thus, the degree of comminution can be adequately determined. (See Fig. 1-2.) It also permits a more accurate reduc-

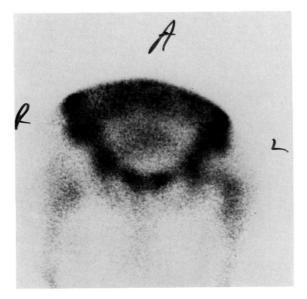

Fig. 1-4. Technetium 99m SC scan of pelvis with subcapital fracture of right hip. Activity absent in region of neck and head of femur on right.

tion, since the capsule is opened. The posterior approach facilitates the addition of supplemental iliac bone. The pedicle graft is secured by inserting the cephalad end into an opening in the femoral head and a screw in the caudal end of the graft. Fracture stability is provided by this additional fixation. Finally, the procedure provides an additional source of blood to the head fragment when the blood supply is diminished or totally absent.

DISADVANTAGES

There are certain disadvantages. However, the disadvantages are not serious enough to preclude using this procedure. The muscle pedicle graft requires a greater degree of technical skill, approximately 30 minutes of increased surgical time as compared to blind nailing, and an increased risk of infection due to greater soft dissection and invasion of the hip joint.

TECHNICAL CONSIDERATIONS

It is generally accepted that the following are principles of surgery for a displaced femoral neck fracture:
1. An accurate reduction must be obtained.
2. The fragment must be impacted.
3. Firm fixation is essential.
The reported experience of many surgeons interested in this fracture has proven this concept. The muscle pedicle graft technique has been adequately described previously.[4,5]

An accurate reduction does not require vigorous manipulation or complicated maneuvers. Manual traction and internal rotation usually are effective in reducing the fracture. Where the fracture is incompletely reduced, a final reduc-

tion can be accomplished under direct vision after opening the capsule.

Impaction of the fragments is accomplished by tightening the nut against the washer at the end of each nail, similar to the tightening procedure on the lugs of a tire wheel.

Firm fixation requires satisfactory placement of four modified Hagie nails (Fig. 1-5). The nails must be placed in the posterior one half and the inferior one half of the femoral head and come to rest no less than 3 mm from the subchondral surface of the femoral head (Fig. 1-6). The direction of the compression force on the femoral head forces the head to rotate posteriorly and inferiorly. The recommended nail placement acts as a neutralization force. The subchondral surface of the head fragment (the only area of compact trabeculae in the osteoporotic head) is the only available area for the fixative to anchor into firm bone. The sparse trabeculation in the intramedullary portions of the neck and head fragments is not conducive to firm fixation of the nails.

RESULTS

The surgical technique used presently was standarized in July of 1971. A total of 253 surgeries have been done, 144 since July, 1971, with a nonunion rate of 9% and 5% respectively. Late segmental collapse has occurred in 5% of the cases.

Results of treatment of displaced subcapital femoral neck fractures in patients under the age of 40 have been discouraging.[8] In this series there were 23 patients in the young adult group. Only one did not unite, and there has been no case with late segmental collapse. In a series of 32 undisplaced fractures or minimally displaced frac-

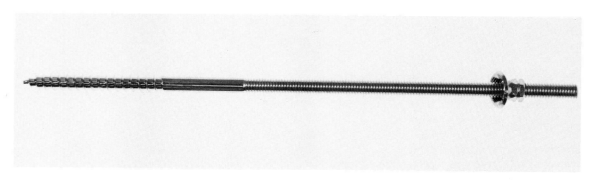

Fig. 1-5. Modified Hagie pin, ³/₁₆ inch (0.5 cm) thick with washer and nut; 1¼ inches (3.1 cm) of cancellous threads.

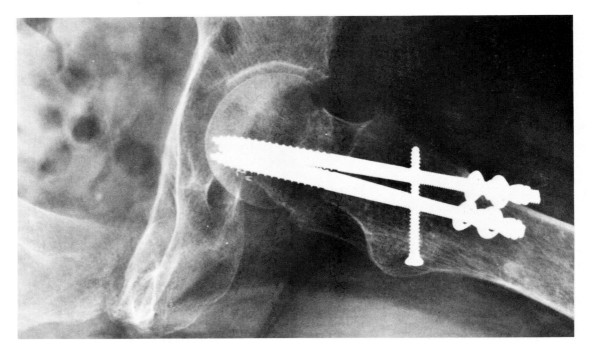

Fig. 1-6. Proper pin placement in posterior one half of head and neck. Pins are up to subchondral bone. Note viable pedicle graft in this healed fracture.

tures (Garden I and II), all have united without any instances of late segmental collapse. Two have had muscle pedicle grafts based on a negative technetium 99m SC hip scan.

CONCLUSION

The importance of strict adherence to the proven principles of accurate reduction, impaction, and rigid fixation in the treatment of displaced femoral neck fractures is to be emphasized. Additionally, the quadratus femoris muscle transplant and autogenous iliac bone chips to fill any defect that may be present in the posterior aspect of the neck are probably necessary to achieve the best results.

The technetium 99m SC bone scan is an important test to assess the status of circulation in the head fragment in undisplaced or minimally displaced fractures. A negative scan indicates severely impaired circulation and the need for a muscle pedicle graft.

REFERENCES

1. Callandruccio, R. A.: The use of radioactive phosporous to determine the viability of the femoral head. In Reynolds, F. C., editor: Proceedings of the Conference on Aseptic Necrosis of the Femoral Head, St. Louis, 1964, Bardgett.

2. Catto, M.: A histological study of avascular necrosis of the femoral head after transcervical fracture, J. Bone Joint Surg. **47-B:**749, 1965.

3. Judet, R.: Traitment des fractures du col du femur par greffe pediculee, Acta Orthop. Scand. **32:**421, 1962.

4. Meyers, M. H., Harvey, J. P., Jr., and Moore, T. M.: Treatment of displaced subcapital and transcervical fractures of the femoral neck by muscle-pedicle bone graft and internal fixation, J. Bone Joint Surg. **55-A:**257, 1973.

5. Meyers, M. H., Harvey, J. P., Jr., and Moore, T. M.: The muscle-pedicle-bone graft in the treatment of displaced fractures of the femoral neck, indications, operative technique, and results, Orthop. Clin. North Am. **5:**779, 1974.

6. Meyers, M. H., Moore, T. M., and Harvey, J. P., Jr.: Displaced fracture of the femoral neck treated with a muscle-pedicle-graft. With emphasis on the treatment of these fractures in young adults, J. Bone Joint Surg. **57-A:**718, 1975.

7. Meyers, M. H., Telfer, N., and Moore, T. M.: Determination of the vascularity of the femoral head with technetium 99m-sulphur-colloid. Diagnostic and prognostic significance, J. Bone Joint Surg. **59-A:**658, 1977.

8. Protzman, R. R., Burkhalter, W. E.: Femoral neck fractures in young adults, J. Bone Joint Surg. **56-A:**1306, 1974.

9. Sevitt, S.: Avascular necrosis and revascularization of the femoral head after intracapsular fractures. A combined arteriographic and histological necropsy study, J. Bone Joint Surg. **46-B:**270, 1964.

Part III

Total hip arthroplasty in acute femoral neck fractures

FRANKLIN H. SIM
RICHARD N. STAUFFER

The displaced intracapsular hip fracture continues to be difficult to manage. Despite significant advances in techniques of internal fixation, the incidences of nonunion and avascular necrosis remain high.[2,36] As a result, prosthetic replacement has been advocated as a solution to this problem.[18]

Although bone union with a viable head is a preferable goal, most physicians agree that prosthetic replacement is indicated for some acute displaced femoral neck fractures.* The questions remain: for whom and under which conditions?

More recently, the question of which type of surgery should be advocated has added further controversy: should it be a hemiarthroplasty or total joint replacement? Previously, the issue of prosthetic replacement was tempered by the realization that functional capacity after insertion of an endoprosthesis was inferior to functional capacity after successful union without necrosis.[25-27] However, the improved functional results and greater predictability of total joint replacement may broaden the indications for replacement surgery in displaced femoral neck fractures.

Criteria for the management of these fractures by internal fixation, hemiarthroplasty, or total hip replacement have not been well-defined.† The three variables, when prosthetic replacement is considered, are the surgeon, the characteristics of the fracture, and the patient.

SURGICAL BIAS

Technical factors are a consideration. Certainly the easiest method of treatment is to insert a prosthesis. Moreover, the surgeon may have a negative attitude about the results of internal fixation. Hargadon and Pearson[22] reported a total failure rate in their series of about 50%. In McNeur's study[35] of 68 displaced fractures of the femoral

*See references 3, 5, 6, 12, 19, 22-24, 33, 34, 37, 40, and 45.
†See references 10, 13-15, 28-30, 32, 35, 37, 38, 41-43, and 46.

neck treated by internal fixation, only 34% were satisfactory, with no significant complications after 2 years. Boyd and Salvatore[9] reported a success rate of 66% in 160 displaced femoral neck fractures. The surgeon may wonder if it is worth subjecting elderly people to a procedure with a chance of ultimate failure of up to 50%.

CONSIDERATIONS OF THE PATIENT

Replacement arthroplasty is of great value in treating the patient rather than in treating the fracture.[31] Physiologic age is only a relative indication. The older the patient and the less cooperation because of senility and neuromuscular disease, the less likely the prolonged nonweight bearing necessary after reduction and fixation will be tolerated. However, Abrami and Stevens[1] did not find that early weight bearing was detrimental to a good result after internal fixation. In addition, it has been shown that age in itself does not predispose either to nonunion or to avascular necrosis in fractures. In Garden's series[20,21] of 60 displaced subcapital fractures and Fielding's series[17,18] of 100 cases, the rate of nonunion was actually highest in the fifth decade. Associated medical conditions and neuromuscular disorders such as Parkinson's disease may encourage prosthetic replacement. In addition, one must consider hip replacement in the displaced intracapsular fracture associated with preexisting symptomatic joint disease, such as degenerative disease, rheumatoid arthritis,[47] or Paget's disease.[44] Although prosthetic replacement might be indicated in certain types of fractures in patients with joint disease, an effort must be made to identify the high-risk fracture in which prosthetic replacement would be advantageous.

CHARACTERISTICS OF THE FRACTURE

Factors affecting the outcome of internal fixation are the level of the fracture, the degree of displacement, and comminution. The incidence of complications is higher in high subcapital fractures. Although these are the most difficult to reduce, they heal satisfactorily when treated by correct reduction and internal fixation. However, the incidence of avascular necrosis is affected by the level of the fracture. Although only 1 of 35 subcapital fractures in Fielding's series[17,18] failed to unite after internal fixation, the rate of avascular necrosis was significantly higher in this group. The degree of displacement seems to be the most important factor in predicting an unsuccessful outcome. In Garden's series,[20,21] the rates of nonunion varied as widely as 7% and 43%. Barnes et al.[4] reporting on 1503 subcapital fractures, had union in all Garden I (incomplete fracture) and II (complete fracture without displacement) fractures and in 67% of Type III (complete fracture with partial displacement) and IV (complete fracture with full displacement) fractures, of which only 14.5% were united at 6 months. Although the degree of displacement did

not adversely affect the rate of union in Fielding's series, the incidence of avascular necrosis was significantly higher in the Garden Type IV fractures. Comminution is a significant factor, not only because of its effect on the retinacular vessels but also because it may prevent a stable reduction.[41,42] Inadequate or incomplete reduction in elderly persons is a relevant indication for prosthetic replacement.

Having addressed the questions of which type of patient and which type of fracture are suitable

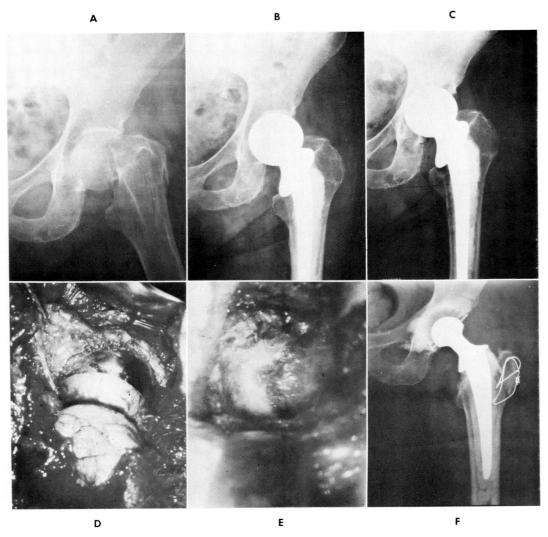

A   B   C

D   E   F

Fig. 1-7. Anteroposterior views and surgical photographs of left hip. **A,** Displaced Garden Type IV subcapital fracture in 78-year-old woman. **B,** Cemented Thompson prosthesis 3 months after operation. **C,** Joint narrowing and erosion of acetabulum 26 months after operation. **D** and **E,** Revision to total hip replacement. Extensive erosion of acetabulum is apparent. **F,** After revision to total hip arthroplasty.

for prosthetic replacement, one must also consider the type of replacement surgery that should be carried out. Is there a place for total hip arthroplasty in acute fractures of the hip, or should a cemented endoprosthesis be used?

ENDOPROSTHETIC REPLACEMENT

Beckenbaugh, Tressler, and Johnson[8] reported on 109 cemented hemiarthroplasties performed at the Mayo Clinic between January, 1969, and December, 1971. (In the same period, 2500 total hip arthroplasties were performed at this institution.) Eighty-eight percent of the patients sustained fractures of the femoral neck or complications thereof. Fifty-one of them, or one half the group, had sustained fresh fractures. In the overall group, one of the major complications was a high rate of infection (4½% compared with 1% in the overall total hip arthro-

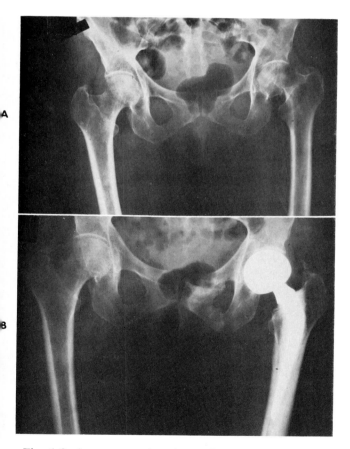

Fig. 1-8. Anteroposterior views of pelvis. **A,** Displaced intracapsular fracture of left hip. **B,** After Bateman endoprosthetic replacement.

plasty series).[7,13] Moreover, reoperations were numerous, accounting for 20% of cases during a 3-year follow-up period.

Review of the 51 hips in 50 patients with cemented endoprostheses for acute femoral neck fractures showed that the fractures were generally displaced high cervical fractures and that replacement surgery was elected because of anticipated high rates of avascular necrosis and nonunion and an inability to control protected ambulation after surgical treatment. Seventeen patients in this group died within the average 36-month follow-up period, but only 3 died in the postoperative period. One patient had a cardiac arrest that was thought to be related to the use of methyl methacrylate. Of the 34 endoprostheses in surviving patients, 4 were frank failures because of pain and were converted to total hip arthroplasties. The patients requiring conversion were active elderly persons in whom erosion through the acetabular cartilage developed quickly, causing pain (Fig. 1-7). Although 85% of the patients had little or no pain, more than half the patients in whom the operation was successful were limited in their activities by nonambulatory existence in nursing homes. This procedure was expedient and successful in providing limited ambulation and absence of pain after hip fracture, but the outcome was unpredictable in previously active patients.

Cabanela and Van Demark[11] reviewed the results in 100 patients who had had a Bateman endoprosthetic procedure performed at the Mayo Clinic since 1974 (Fig. 1-8). This procedure was used to treat 58 patients with acute femoral neck fractures. There were 48 women and 10 men from 49 to 96 years of age (average, 79.4 years). Eight patients in this group died, three in the postoperative period. There were two dislocations and one superficial infection. Twenty-three patients were available for follow-up for between 12 and 40 months (average, 20 months); the results were graded as excellent in 10, good in 8, fair in 4, and poor in 1.

TOTAL HIP ARTHROPLASTY

Between 1970 and 1978, 112 patients (19 men and 93 women) at the Mayo Clinic had a total hip arthroplasty for acute femoral neck fractures. The median age was 74 years (range, 40 to 89 years). Length of follow-up by clinical and roentgenographic examinations for 110 patients was from 9 days to 7 years (median, 1½ years). The average interval between injury and surgery was 2½ days. This delay reflected the time necessary to evaluate and treat the many medical problems in this elderly group of patients. Sixty percent of this group had a physical status rating of 3 or greater according to the classification of the American Society of Anesthesiology,[16] an indication of severe systemic disturbance such as a severely limiting organic disease. Pre-existing medical problems were present in 74 patients (67%), including serious cardiovascular, pulmonary, or renal disorders. In addition, 5 patients had pre-existing neoplastic conditions that did not involve the hip; because of their previous level of activity and shortened life expectancy, it was thought

that these patients would benefit from the functional restoration afforded by total joint replacement.

Roentgenograms showed that all the fractures were displaced; 60 (53.5%) were classified as Garden Type IV, 39 (34.8%) as Type III, and 13 (11.6%) as Type II. Seventy-one of the fractures (63.3%) were subcapital; 31 (27.6%) were midcervical, and 10 (8.9%) were basilar. The acetabulum was considered normal in 57 patients, with slight narrowing in 30, moderate degeneration in 17, and severe degeneration in 6. Of those with acetabular disease, 8 had symptomatic degenerative joint disease (Fig. 1-9), 5 had rheumatoid arthritis (Fig. 1-10), and 3 had Paget's disease (Fig. 1-11). Significant osteoporosis were present in 74

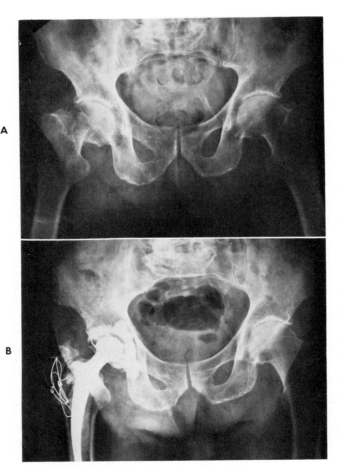

Fig. 1-9. Anteroposterior views of pelvis. **A,** Displaced intracapsular fracture of right hip with associated symptomatic degenerative joint disease. **B,** Three months after total hip replacement.

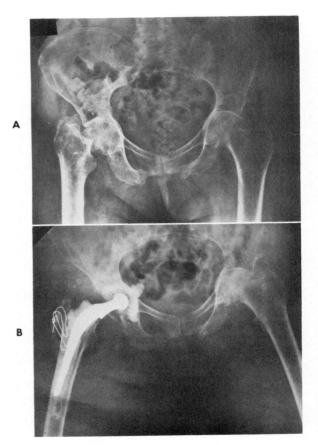

Fig. 1-10. Anteroposterior views of pelvis. **A,** Displaced intracapsular fracture of right hip with associated rheumatoid arthritis. **B,** Three months after total hip replacement.

patients (67%). Contralateral hip disease was noted in nine patients (Fig. 1-12).

Results

Five kinds of total hip arthroplasty were used, with the Charnley prosthesis selected for more than one half the cases. The trochanter was removed through a straight lateral approach in 62 cases; in the rest, a posterior or anterior approach was used. The average surgical time was 116 minutes, with an anesthesia time of 180 minutes. In comparison, the average anesthesia time in the cemented hemiarthroplasty series was 168 minutes.[8] The average blood replacement was 2.5 units as compared to 1.5 units in the hemiarthroplasty group. Full weight bearing was encouraged as tolerated in the group without trochanteric osteotomies but was delayed 6 weeks in the others. The average length of time in the hospital was 22 days.

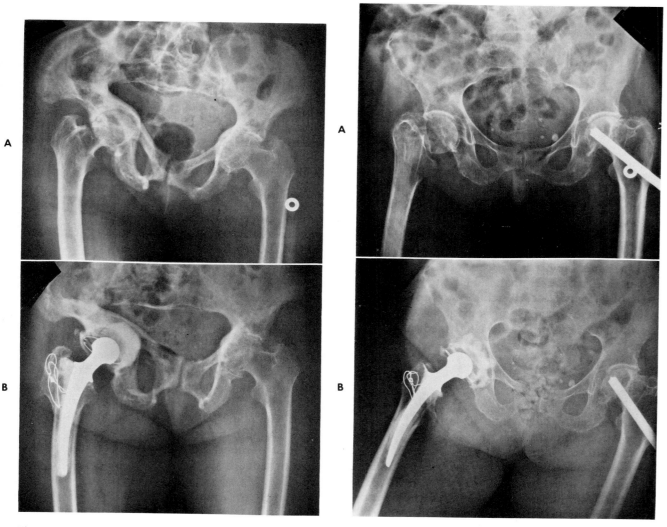

Fig. 1-11. Anteroposterior views of pelvis in 76-year-old woman with Paget's disease. **A,** Associated fracture of right femoral neck. **B,** Twenty-one months after total hip arthroplasty.

Fig. 1-12. Anteroposterior views of pelvis in 88-year-old woman. **A,** Displaced intracapsular fracture of right hip. Patient also has incapacitating symptoms due to avascular necrosis of contralateral hip. **B,** One month after total hip replacement.

Twenty patients died during the follow-up period. Only one of the deaths occurred during hospitalization for the procedure. None of the delayed deaths was related to the operation or the fracture. Of 85 patients evaluated after 1 year, 69 (81.2%) had no pain, and 15 (17.6%) had mild discomfort. In one patient, the pain was judged to be moderate. After operation, the range of motion was recorded in 100 patients. The range was 100 degrees or more in 47 patients and more than 90 degrees in 45. Only 8 patients had less than 90 degrees of motion. These results compare favorably with those of our overall series of total hip replacements. Leg lengths, measured after operation in 89 patients, were equal in 74 (83%). Four patients had a discrepancy of more than 0.5 inch (1.27 cm).

The state of activity and use of assistive devices varied with the preoperative status of the patient. Before the injury, 79 patients were unrestricted or mildly restricted in their activity; 25 were moderately restricted, and 6 had severe restriction. Of the 35 patients who used assistive devices for ambulation before operation, 26 had a cane, 4 had crutches, and 3 had a walker. In addition, 2 patients were unable to walk.

After the operation, activity was not restricted or was mildly restricted in 62 patients, was moderately restricted in 30, and was severely restricted in 9. Fifty-five used assistive devices: 43 used a cane, 4 used crutches, and 8 used a walker. Most patients maintained their previous levels of activity, but 13 actually improved, and 33 were worse. Decrease in activity was generally due to deterioration in associated medical conditions.

Roentgenographic findings

Roentgenograms made at an average of 22 months after the operation were reviewed for 95 patients. A slight lucent line of less than 1 mm was noted around the femoral component in 7% and around the acetabular component in 8%. One patient had resorption of the medial calcar. Heterotopic bone formation was mild in 10 patients and pronounced in 2 others. Of the 62 patients on which a trochanteric osteotomy was performed, 50 had in situ healing; 3 had migratory healing, and 3 had nonunion. In 6 patients, broken trochanteric wires were visible on roentgenograms.

Complications

Of 112 patients, 21% had medical complications. Clinical phlebitis was diagnosed in 1 patient, and 5 patients had pulmonary embolism. Seven patients had cardiac, 7 had renal, and 4 had gastrointestinal complications that were significant. The only instance of postoperative infection was superficial and was responsive to local debridement and antibiotics. The rate of infection compared favorably with the 0.9% in our overall series of total hip arthroplasties and contrasts with the 4.1% in the group of cemented hemiarthroplasties.

Wound hematomas, one requiring drainage, occurred in 5 patients. Significant heterotopic bone formation was noted in 2 patients, and 3 patients had complications related to the trochanteric osteotomy. Dislocations occurred in 12 patients; thus, the rate was high. Ten were successfully treated by closed reduction; one patient had recurrent dislocation that remains unreduced, and another patient required open reduction 4 months after the operation. Nerve injuries developed in 2 patients after the operation, one a peroneal nerve injury and the other a sciatic palsy. Four patients required additional surgery. The procedures performed were debridement of a superficial infection, evacuation of a hematoma, open reduction of a dislocation, and reattachment of the trochanter. The patient requiring the latter procedure also had removal of heterotopic bone.

COMMENT

Efforts are being made to better define the role of replacement arthroplasty in the treatment of acute femoral neck fractures. If replacement is indicated, should a cemented endoprosthesis or perhaps a Bateman prosthesis be used, or is there a place for total hip arthroplasty? We concluded from analyzing our results that the primary indication for the cemented endoprosthesis is a fresh femoral neck fracture in a minimally active or nonambulatory elderly patient with osteoporosis. A Bateman endoprosthesis may be considered for a fairly inactive elderly patient with a displaced subcapital fracture and a normal acetabulum who can be expected to resume some limited activity. In the previously active elderly patient who meets the criteria for prosthetic replacement, total hip arthroplasty is preferred.

There is considerable agreement about the use of total hip arthroplasty for complications (such as avascular necrosis, delayed union, and non-union) of femoral neck fractures treated by internal fixation, particularly if there is loss of articular cartilage in the acetabulum.[25-27] Also, total hip arthroplasty may be indicated after endoprostheses have failed in acute fractures.

In addition, total hip arthroplasty was considered for 16 patients because of associated hip disease. Until recently, the problem of fracture of the femoral neck associated with Paget's disease was considered to be unsolved, with a pessimistic outlook after internal fixation or prosthetic replacement. Our experience to date with total hip arthroplasty appears to offer a solution to this problem.[44] Moreover, in 9 patients in this series, associated contralateral hip disease was a factor in selection for total hip arthroplasty.

Results in our series indicate that total hip arthroplasty has a definite place in properly selected patients with acute femoral neck fractures. However, the selection of these patients remains a challenge to the judgment of the surgeon. A significant number of active elderly patients in this series exibited associated medical conditions that were thought to preclude a second operation because of increased risk. As the popularity of total hip arthroplasty for a variety of disorders increases, one must certainly observe caution with its use in patients with acute fractures. Valuable as the prosthesis is, it is never as good as the patient's own hip. We must also consider the morbidity of this procedure in patients of advanced age.[39] In our series, 21% had postoperative medical complications, and 22% had surgical complications. With the widespread use of total hip arthroplasty as the primary treatment for femoral neck fractures, one might expect morbidity to increase to unacceptable levels. We believe that this procedure is best reserved for active elderly patients with fractures in which standard internal fixation is likely to fail or with significant pre-existing hip disease.

REFERENCES

1. Abrami, G., and Stevens, J: Early weight bearing after internal fixation of transcervical fracture of the femur: preliminary report of a clinical trial, J. Bone Joint Surg. **46-B:**204, 1964.
2. Albright, J. P.: Treatment for fixation complications: femoral neck fractures, Arch. Surg. **110:**30, 1975.
3. Anderson, L. D., Hamsa, W. R., Jr., and Waring, T. L.: Femoral-head prostheses: a review of three hundred and fifty-six operations and their results, J. Bone Joint Surg. **46-A:**1049, 1964.
4. Barnes, R., Brown, J. T., Garden, R. S., and Nicoll, E. A.: Subcapital fractures of the femur: a prospective review, J. Bone Joint Surg. **58-B:**2, 1976.
5. Barr, J. S., Compere, E. L., Ghormley, R. K., Jergesen, F. H., Preston, R. L., and Thomson, J. E. M.: A symposium on hip joint prostheses. In American Academy of Orthopaediac Surgeons: Instructional course lectures, vol. 15, St. Louis, 1958, The C. V. Mosby Co., p. 1.
6. Barr, J. S., Donovan, J. F., and Florence, D. W.: Arthroplasty of the hip: theoretical and practical considerations with a follow-up study of prosthetic replacement of the femoral head at the Massachusetts General Hospital, J. Bone Joint Surg. **46-A:**249, 1964.
7. Beckenbaugh, R. D., and Ilstrup, D. M.: Total hip arthroplasty: a review of three hundred and thirty-three cases with long follow-up, J. Bone Joint Surg. **60-A:**306, 1978.
8. Beckenbaugh, R. D., Tressler, H. A., and Johnson, E. W., Jr.: Results after hemiarthroplasty of the hip using a cemented femoral prosthesis: a review of 109 cases with an average follow-up of 36 months, Mayo Clin. Proc. **52:**349, 1977.
9. Boyd, H. B., and Salvatore, J. E.: Acute fracture of the femoral neck: internal fixation or prosthesis? J. Bone Joint Surg. **46-A:**1066, 1964.
10. Bradford, C. H., Kelleher, J. J., O'Brien, P. I., and Kilfoyle, R. M.: Primary prosthesis for subcapital fractures of the neck of the femur: preliminary report, N. Engl. J. Med. **251:**804, 1954.
11. Cabanela, M. E., and Van Demark, R. E., Jr.: Presented at American Orthopaedic Society Annual Meeting, June 16 to 19, 1980, Hawaii.
12. Carnesale, P. G., and Anderson, L. D.: Primary prosthetic replacement for femoral neck fractures, Arch. Surg. **110:**27, 1975.
13. Coventry, M. B.: Fresh fracture of the hip treated with prosthesis. In American Academy of Orthopaedic Surgeons: Instructional course lectures, vol. 16, St. Louis, 1959, The C. V. Mosby Co., p. 292.
14. D'Arcy, J., and Devas, M.: Treatment of fractures of the femoral neck by replacement with the Thompson prosthesis, J. Bone Joint Surg. **58-8:**279, 1976.
15. Deyerle, W. M.: Multiple-pin peripheral fixation in fractures of the neck of the femur: immediate weight bearing, Clin. Orthop. **39:**135, 1965.
16. Dripps, R. D., Eckenhoff, J. E., and Vandam, L. D.: Introduction to anesthesia: the principles of safe practice, ed. 4, Philadelphia, 1972, W. B. Saunders Co.
17. Fielding, J.: Displaced femoral neck fractures, Orthop. Rev. **2:**11, 1973.
18. Fielding, J. W., Wilson, S. A., and Ratzan, S.: A continuing end-result study of displaced intracapsular fractures of the neck of the femur treated with the Pugh nail, J. Bone Joint Surg. **56-A:**1464, 1974.
19. Ford, L. T., and Key, A. J.: Replacement prosthesis for fractures of the neck of the femur, J. Iowa State Med. Soc. **45:**597, 1955.

20. Garden, R. S.: Low-angle fixation in fractures of the femoral neck, J. Bone Joint Surg. **43-B:**647, 1961.
21. Garden, R. S.: Stability and union in subcapital fractures of the femur, J. Bone Joint Surg. **46-B:**630, 1964.
22. Hargadon, E. J., and Pearson, J. R.: Treatment of intracapsular fractures of the femoral neck with the Charnley compression screw, J. Bone Joint Surg. **45-B:**305, 1963.
23. Hinchey, J. J.: An evaluation of prosthetic replacement in management of fresh fractures of the neck of the femur. In American Academy of Orthopaedic Surgeons: Instructional course lectures, vol. 17, St. Louis, 1960, The C. V. Mosby Co., p. 121.
24. Hinchey, J. J., and Day, P. L.: Primary prosthetic replacement in fresh femoral-neck fractures: a review of 294 consecutive cases, J. Bone Joint Surg. **46:**223, 1964.
25. Hunter, G.: Treatment of fractures of the neck of the femur, Can. Med. Assoc. J. **117:**60, 1977.
26. Hunter, G. A.: A comparison of the use of internal fixation and prosthetic replacement for fresh fractures of the neck of the femur, Br. J. Surg. **56:**229, 1969.
27. Hunter, G. A.: A further comparison of the use of internal fixation and prosthetic replacement for fresh fractures of the neck of the femur, Br. J. Surg. **61:**382, 1974.
28. Jensen, J. S., and Holstein, P.: A long-term follow-up of Moore arthroplasty in femoral neck fractures, Acta Orthop. Scand. **46:**764, 1975.
29. Johnson, J. T. H., and Crothers, O.: Nailing versus prosthesis for femoral-neck fractures: a critical review of long-term results in two hundred and thirty-nine consecutive private patients, J. Bone Joint Surg. **57-A:**686, 1975.
30. Lindholm, R. V., Puranen, J., and Kinnunen, P.: The Moore Vitallium femoral-head prosthesis in fractures of the femoral neck, Acta Orthop. Scand. **47:**70, 1976.
31. Lunceford, E. M., Jr.: Use of the Moore self-locking Vitallium prosthesis in acute fractures of the femoral neck, J. Bone Joint Surg. **47-A:**832, 1965.
32. Lunt, H. R. W.: The role of prosthetic replacement of the head of the femur as primary treatment for subcapital fractures, Injury **3:**107, 1971.
33. Mahoney, J. W., Mulholland, J. H., Jahr, J., and Dooling, J. A.: Immediate Moore prosthetic replacement in acute intracapsular fractures. Am. J. Surg. **95:**577, 1958.
34. McElvenny, R. T.: Concepts and principles in the treatment of intracapsular fractures of the hip, Am. J. Orthop. **2:**161, 1960.
35. McNeur, J. C.: The treatment of subcapital fractures of the neck of the femur with a nail-plate and wedge osteotomy, J. Bone Joint Surg. **35-B:**188, 1953.
36. Meyers, M. H., Harvey, J. P., Jr., and Moore, T. M.: Treatment of displaced subcapital and transcervical fractures of the femoral neck by muscle-pedicle-bone graft and internal fixation, J. Bone Joint Surg. **55-A:**257, 1973.
37. Nicoll, E. A.: The unsolved fracture (editorial), J. Bone Joint Surg. **45-B:**239, 1963.
38. Raine, G. E. T.: A comparison of internal fixation and prosthetic replacement for recent displaced subcapital fractures of the neck of the femur, Injury **5:**25, 1973.
39. Reno, J. H., and Burlington, H.: Fractures of the hip—a mortality survey, Am. J. Surg. **95:**581, 1958.
40. Salvati, E. A., and Wilson, P. D., Jr.: Long-term results of femoral-head replacement, J. Bone Joint Surg. **55-A:**516, 1973.
41. Scheck, M.: Intracapsular fractures of the femoral neck: comminution of the posterior neck cortex as a cause of unstable fixation, J. Bone Joint Surg. **41-A:**1187, 1959.
42. Scheck, M.: Management of fractures of the femoral neck, J. Bone Joint Surg. **47-A:**819, 1965.
43. Søreide, O., Lerner, A. P., and Thunold, J.: Primary prosthetic replacement in acute femoral neck fractures, Injury **6:**286, 1975.
44. Stauffer, R. N., and Sim, F. H.: Total hip arthroplasty in Paget's disease of the hip, J. Bone Joint Surg. **58-A:**476, 1976.
45. Thompson, F. R.: Two and a half years' experience with a Vitallium intramedullary hip prosthesis, J. Bone Joint Surg. **36A:**489, 1954.
46. Tillberg, B.: Treatment of fractures of the femoral neck by primary arthroplasty, Acta Orthop. Scand. **47:**209, 1976.
47. Vahvanen, V.: Femoral neck fracture of the rheumatoid hip joint: a study of 20 operatively treated cases, Acta Rheum. Scand. **17:**125, 1971.

Chapter 2

Condylocephalic nailing of intertrochanteric and subtrochanteric fractures of the femur

Part I

Closed intramedullary nailing of intertrochanteric and subtrochanteric fractures of the femur

LESLIE J. HARRIS

The primary goal in the treatment of patients with intertrochanteric fractures is to minimize patient mortality. Despite the improvement of fixation devices used for intertrochanteric fractures over the past 50 years, early postoperative mortality rates are 12% to 16%, and late mortality rates may vary from 20% to 42%.* The operative trauma to these often debilitated geriatric patients should, therefore, be minimized. Furthermore, since many of these patients are unable to follow a postoperative program of nonweight bearing on their injured extremities, the fixation must be adequate to permit immediate weight bearing. Condylocephalic nailing is a closed procedure that is minimally invasive. Moreover, the orientation of the nail is mechanically efficient and allows early weight bearing for patients with intertrochanteric fractures and for many patients with subtrochanteric fractures.

HISTORICAL REVIEW

In 1966, Kuntscher[14] described "condylocephalic nailing" of intertrochanteric fractures. The implant is a modification of a nail previously described by Lezius[15] and is inserted over a guide

pin from the medial femoral condyle, up the medullary canal, and into the femoral head. In 1970, Ender reported a technique that was a further modification of Kuntscher's procedure. Three or four smooth pins are inserted above the medial epicondyle into the medullary canal of the femur to diverge into the femoral head.[13] The greater curvature and flexibility of the Ender pins, compared to the Kuntscher nail, facilitates their placement in the femoral head. Complications reported with the use of Kuntscher's and Ender's techniques include (1) penetration of the femoral head (2) postoperative distal migration of the nail interfering with knee function, and (3) external rotation deformity.[8,9,13]

DESIGN CONSIDERATIONS

In 1973 we began an investigation into the condylocephalic nailing procedure and examined possible changes in the implant and instrumentation that would simplify the surgical technique and lower the incidence of the reported complications. The intramedullary nail that has evolved is a single, solid nail with a diamond-shaped cross section. When in situ, the proximal portion of the nail is at an angle of approximately 160 degrees to the femoral shaft in the frontal plane (Fig. 2-1). The nail is, therefore, aligned approximately parallel to average loading forces on the proximal femur, and bending moments acting on the implant are minimized.[11,16,21] The nail is contoured in the lateral plane to incorporate a 10-degree anteroposterior bow and an 8-degree anteversion curvature (Fig. 2-1). The nail is manufactured from titanium 6-aluminum 4-vanadium (Ti-6-4). This alloy has superior yield and fatigue strengths and approximately one half the modu-

---

*See references 6, 7, 10, 17-19, and 22.

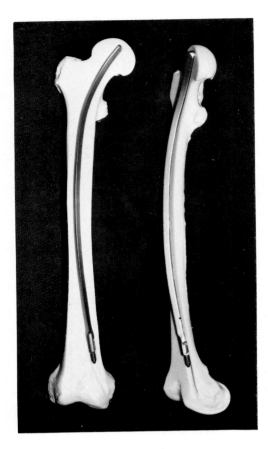

Fig. 2-1. Frontal and oblique views of condylocephalic nail in femoral models. In the frontal plane the proximal portion of the nail is aligned approximately 160 degrees to the femoral shaft. In the lateral plane the nail incorporates a 10-degree anteroposterior bow and an 8-degree anteversion angle. Distal end of the nail should lie 2 to 4 cm within the medullary canal.

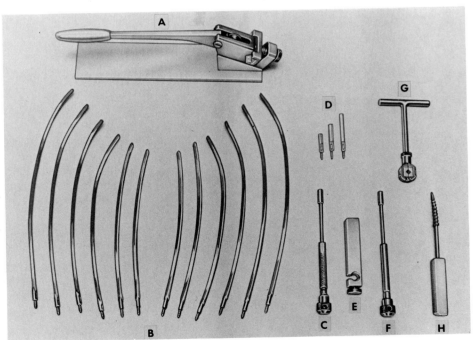

Fig. 2-2. Nails and instrumentation. **A,** Nail bending device. **B,** Left and right nails 32 to 48 cm in length. **C,** Driver-extractor used with nail extenders (reverse threaded). **D,** Nail extenders 3 to 7 cm in length. **E,** Extractor bar. **F,** Driver-extractor used with nails. **G,** Rotational guide. **H,** Broach.

lus of elasticity of 316L stainless steel and cobalt-chromium alloys.* When similar structural designs are compared, the Ti-6-4 alloy provides less rigid fracture fixation than implants of the latter two alloys. Considerable experimental work with bone plates and, more recently, with intramedullary rods suggests that low modulus implants reduce the deleterious effects of stress shielding on fracture repair and bone remodeling and may result in mechanically stronger fracture healing.† Furthermore, the relative elasticity of the implant facilitates the actual intramedullary nailing procedure.

Instrumentation includes left and right nails of various lengths, nail extenders, driver extractors, a nail rotational guide, a broach, and a nail bending device (Fig. 2-2).

INDICATIONS AND CONTRAINDICATIONS

Preliminary indications for condylocephalic nailing have included the following fractures in adult patients: intertrochanteric and subtrochanteric fractures, ipsilateral shaft intertrochanteric

---

*Zimmer U.S.A. Materials Research Laboratory: Tivanium (titanium 6-aluminum 4-vanadium), Warsaw, Ind., 1978.
†See references 1, 2, 4, 23, and 24.

fractures, and pathologic fractures of the trochanteric region. Relative contraindications include transcervical fractures, obliteration of the medullary canal by previous fracture healing or osteoblastic tumors (e.g., metastatic prostatic carcinoma), medullary canal isthmus diameters less than 11 mm, multiple metastatic lesions of the femoral shaft (e.g., multiple myeloma), and the presence of active infection.

OPERATIVE PROCEDURE

Under spinal or general anesthesia, the patient is positioned supine on the fracture table with the image intensifier located lateral to the involved hip. Traction is applied with the involved lower extremity abducted 20 to 30 degrees and in neutral rotation. The uninvolved lower extremity is maximally abducted to facilitate lateral projections with the image intensifier (Fig. 2-3). The preliminary closed reduction is evaluated in anteroposterior and lateral image intensifier views, and adjustments in traction are made as needed. Often slight flexion and/or external rotation of the leg is required to obtain fracture reduction. The leg is prepared from midtibia to the superior iliac crest. The surgeon is postioned at the medial aspect of the leg, the assistant laterally.

A 2.5 cm longitudinal incision is begun approx-

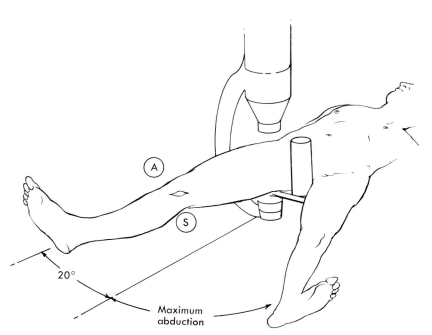

Fig. 2-3. Setup of patient supine on fracture table with image intensifier located lateral to the involved hip. (See text.)

imately 2 cm anterior to the adductor tubercle and continued distally. The incision is carried through the interval between the vastus medialis and adductor magnus over the proximal half of the wound. A hole in the cortex is made in the midcoronal plane of the femur directly anterior to the adductor tubercle, using the special broach. The insertion site is, therefore, located approximately 2 cm anterior to the adductor tubercle, or halfway between the plane of the patella and the adductor tubercle (Fig. 2-4). Care must be taken not to place the insertion site too far posteriorly, which may result in comminution anterior to the cortical hole during the insertion of the appliance.

Selection of the proper nail length is determined by superimposing a nail over the femur with the image intensifier so that its proximal tip overlies the femoral head. Estimation of nail length should take into account that the distal end of the nail should ultimately lie 2 to 4 cm proximal to the insertion site, that is, countersunk to at least 2 cm within the medullary canal. With impaction or telescoping at the fracture site, the nail may then settle distally without impinging on the quadriceps mechanism.

The nail is inserted approximately perpendicular to the femoral shaft and is rapidly brought to an orientation that is nearly parallel to the long axis of the femur as it is driven proximally. The anteroposterior (AP) plane of the nail is aligned with the AP plane of the femur using the T-bar guide; the horizontal part of the T is placed parallel to or in slight external rotation to the plane of the patella (Fig. 2-5). This is most easily visualized with the leg in neutral rotation (patella parallel to floor). It should be remembered that starting the nail in external or internal rotation with respect to the femur causes it to track, anteriorly or posteriorly respectively, in the femoral shaft. If during the procedure it appears that the nail is significantly malrotated with respect to the femoral shaft, it should be withdrawn, realigned, and readvanced. The guide *should not* be used to forcibly rotate the nail within the femoral canal.

The nail is driven up the femoral canal, across the fracture site, and into the proximal fragment a short distance (1 to 3 cm). At this point, the final reduction should be carefully considered. Anteroposterior and lateral image intensifier views are examined, and final adjustments in alignment are made. A valgus reduction should be obtained for all unstable intertrochanteric fractures. To obtain a valgus reposition, the leg is widely abducted as medially directed pressure is applied over the trochanter. The rotatory alignment should be carefully assessed on the lateral view. After the surgeon is entirely satisfied with the position of the fracture fragments, the nail is driven into the proximal fragment to within 5 mm of the subchondral cortex of the femoral head. The traction is then released and the frac-

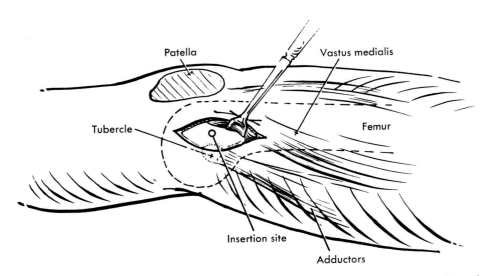

Fig. 2-4. Nail insertion site. The cortical hole is made with the broach approximately midway between medial edge of patella and adductor tubercle.

ture impacted manually. The medial retinaculum is then repaired, the skin closed, and a light compressive dressing applied.

Care should be taken when using the broach, as well as during the nailing procedure itself, to avoid iatrogenic fracturing of the osteoporotic

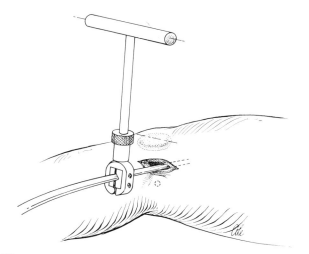

Fig. 2-5. Nail rotational guide. To establish the correct rotation of the nail with respect to the femur, the horizontal part of the T is placed parallel or in slight external rotation to the plane of the patella. The guide should *not* be used to forcibly rotate the nail within the femoral canal.

bone in elderly patients. The nail should advance easily through the medullary canal. If an excessive amount of force is required to advance the nail, the surgeon should evaluate the following potential causes of binding: (1) improper location of the insertion site, (2) poor alignment of the nail with respect to the femur, and (3) possible anatomic anomaly of the femur.

SPECIAL CONSIDERATIONS

Manipulation. Manipulation is occasionally required to negotiate the nail across the fracture site. The shaft fragment may sag posterior to the head-neck fragment as seen in the lateral image intensifier projection. Reduction is achieved by having the assistant lift the thigh anteriorly as the nail is driven into the proximal fragment.

The nail tip may exit from the fracture site medially when nailing intertrochanteric or subtrochanteric fractures with medial displacement of the shaft or extensive medial comminution (Fig. 2-6, *A*). To pass the nail across the fracture site, the physician temporarily places the fracture in a varus position. Simply adducting the leg is often all that is required, but, if necessary, further angulation is accomplished by relaxing the distal traction and applying lateral traction at the fracture site by means of a surgical sheet wrapped around the proximal thigh (Fig. 2-6, *B*). After the nail is 1 to 3 cm beyond the fracture site, the

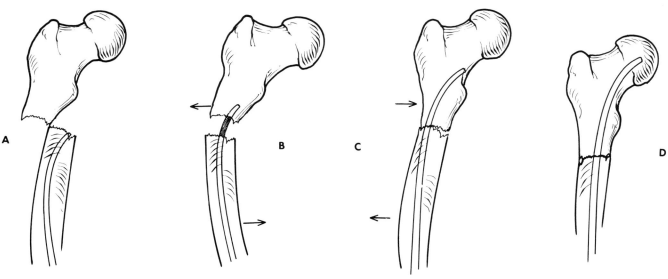

Fig. 2-6. If the nail exits the fracture site medially, manipulation of the leg is required to pass the nail into the proximal fragment. (See text.)

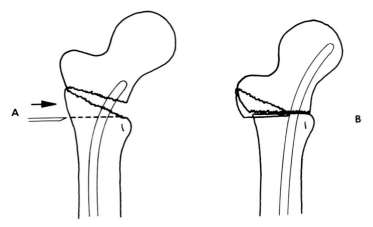

Fig. 2-7. Percutaneous osteotomy of greater trochanter. **A,** The image intensifier is used to localize the position of the osteotome inserted through a small stab incision over the lateral thigh. The osteotomy is ideally done after the nail is 1 to 3 cm across the fracture site. **B,** The leg is abducted, and medially directed pressure is applied over the trochanteric area to obtain valgus alignment with medial displacement of the shaft. This maneuver also allows the nail to be positioned more inferiorly in the femoral head.

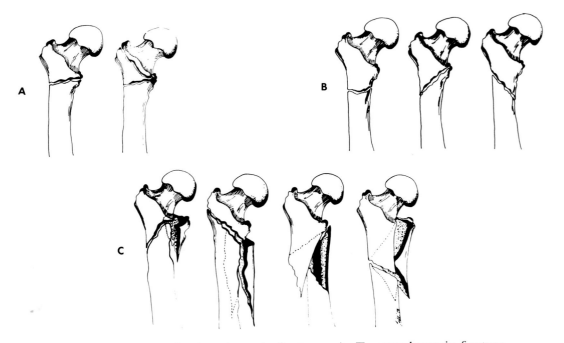

Fig. 2-8. Classifications of subtrochanteric fractures. **A,** Transtrochanteric fracture. Horizontal or slightly oblique fracture at the level of the lesser trochanter with or without extension into the intertrochanteric region. **B,** Stable subtrochanteric fracture. Horizontal or short oblique fracture at a level between the lower margin of the lesser trochanter and 5 cm distally. The major fracture line measures between 90 degrees and 45 degrees to the axis of the femoral shaft. There is no significant posterior or medial comminution. **C,** Unstable subtrochanteric fracture. Horizontal or short oblique fracture with posteromedial comminution or long spiral fractures. The major fracture line of long spiral fractures is angulated less than 45 degrees to the axis of the shaft (usually approximately 30 degrees). These fractures are most often associated with significant comminution.

leg is gradually abducted, and the fracture is reduced in slight valgus position as the nail is driven proximally along the inferior cortex of the femoral neck (Fig. 2-6, *C* and *D*).

Supplemental procedures. Occasionally a supplemental procedure may be required. When valgus positioning of unstable intertrochanteric fractures cannot be obtained by closed manipulation, a percutaneous trochanteric osteotomy as recommended by Bohler[14] should be considered. The image intensifier is used to localize the position of the osteotome inserted through a small stab incision over the lateral thigh. The osteotomy is ideally done after the nail has been driven 1 to 3 cm across the fracture site (Fig. 2-7, *A* and *B*). When attempts at closed nailing of subtrochanteric fractures fail, a small midlateral thigh exposure may be required to guide the nail across the fracture site under direct vision.

Alteration of nail curvature. Preoperative roentgenograms should be carefully examined for anatomic variations such as coxa vara, coxa valga, excessive femoral anteversion, and extreme anteroposterior or varus bowing of the femoral diaphysis. Congenital anomalies may preclude the use of the implant, or under unusual circumstances, the nail may be contoured to fit the patient's anatomy. Alteration of the nail curvature has also been occasionally required for subtochanteric fractures and pathologic lesions that extend into the femoral diaphyseal region. When the nail is straightened slightly in the frontal plane, it is more easily negotiated across defects in the medial cortex of the medullary canal. The straightened nail also facilitates a valgus reduction of subtrochanteric fractures.

POSTOPERATIVE MANAGEMENT

Patients with intertrochanteric, transtrochanteric, and stable subtrochanteric fractures (Fig. 2-8) are encouraged to begin progressive weight-bearing ambulation within the first postoperative week. When ambulation is delayed because of the patient's general condition or other injuries, the leg is placed in an antirotation splint until ambulation is possible. Patients with unstable subtrochanteric fractures are maintained in balanced suspension for 3 to 6 weeks before weight bearing is allowed.

CLINICAL SERIES

Our experience with condylocephalic nailing encompasses approximately 240 intertrochanteric

and subtrochanteric fractures over the past 5 years (Figs. 2-9 to 2-12). The results of treatment of 185 nonpathologic fractures that were followed to radiographic union (minimum 8 months) are summarized here. The follow-up ranged from 8 to 62 months, with a median of 23 months.

Intertrochanteric fractures were considered unstable or stable on the basis of posteromedial comminution as described by Dimon and Hughston.[5] There were 133 intertrochanteric fractures, including 41 unstable and 92 stable fractures. A classification into three subgroups of 52 subtrochanteric fractures were used. (Fig 2-8). There were 21 transtrochanteric, 8 stable subtrochanteric, and 23 unstable subtrochanteric fractures.

The mean age of the 185 patients was 75 (range, 21 to 103 years). The ages of the patients with intertrochanteric and transtrochanteric fractures averaged 78. The average age of those with stable and unstable subtrochanteric fractures was 48 years.

Results

The operative procedure averaged 22 minutes for intertrochanteric and transtrochanteric fractures. Subtrochanteric fractures averaged 65 minutes. All intertrochanteric fractures underwent closed nailings, whereas three of the 52 subtrochanteric fractures required open reduction. Five of the 41 unstable intertrochanteric fractures had percutaneous osteotomies of the greater trochanter to achieve vulgus reductions. Operative blood loss was less than 50 ml in all cases, except the three subtrochanteric fractures, which had open reductions.

The average hospital stay for patients with intertrochanteric fractures was 9.6 days (range, 3 to 29 days) and for those with transtrochanteric fractures, 10.4 days (range, 4 to 21 days). The hospital stay for patients with distal subtrochanteric fractures averaged 28.6 days (range, 6 to 39 days). The variable period of time that walkers, crutches, and canes were used depended mostly on the general physical and mental condition of the patient rather than the type of fracture.

Of 149 patients who were community ambulators (fully ambulatory outside the home) prior to their fractures, 138 regained their prefracture ambulatory status within 6 months. Ten of the sixteen minimally ambulatory patients were bedridden at 6 months follow-up. All of the twenty previously nonambulatory patients remained nonambulatory. Seventy-one percent of the pa-

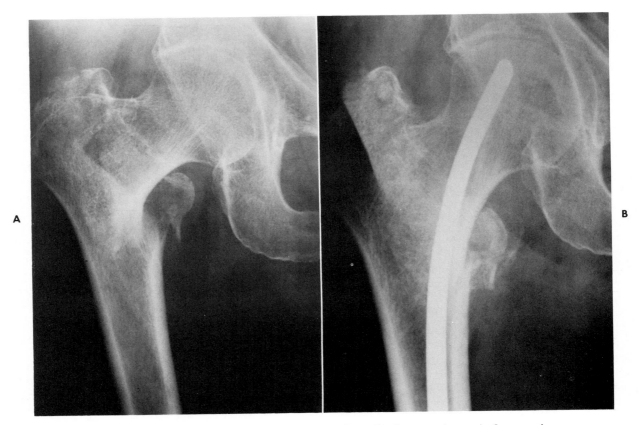

Fig. 2-9. A, Anteroposterior roentgenogram of a stable intertrochanteric fracture in a 58-year-old man. Patient underwent closed intramedullary nailing and began progressive weight-bearing ambulation 2 days after surgery. **B,** Anteroposterior roentgenogram 3 months after surgery. The patient is ambulating without assistive devices and is asymptomatic. Note nail position adjacent to fracture site medially and parallel to the primary trabeculae of the head and neck.

tients were able to begin weight-bearing ambulation within 2 weeks after the operation. Early weight bearing did not appear to disturb fracture alignment. Weight bearing in the twenty-three patients with unstable subtrochanteric fractures was routinely delayed 3 to 6 weeks.

Fracture union was judged by the absence of pain and roentgenographic evidence of mature bone bridging the fracture site. Intertrochanteric and transtrochanteric fractures required an average of 11 weeks for clinical union, while subtrochanteric fractures took an average of 18 weeks.

Changes in leg lengths secondary to fracture impaction, telescoping of fragments, and varus or valgus reductions were assessed by x-ray measurements. Thirty of the 41 unstable intertrochanteric, 5 of the 21 transtrochanteric, and 11 of 23 unstable subtrochanteric fractures had im-

paction or telescoping of 5 to 20 mm, with an average of 11 mm. The maximum of 20 mm shortening occurred in three patients with unstable intertrochanteric fractures.

There were no delayed unions, nonunions, or infections. There were no cases of penetration of the nail through the femoral head; with impaction at the fracture site, the proximal fragment and the nail consistently settled distally as a unit.

Complications and discussion

An examination of orthopaedic complications that have occurred emphasizes important technical considerations as well as relative advantages and disadvantages of this procedure compared to standard open hip nailing techniques.

External rotation deformity. Of 149 ambulatory patients, seven (4.7%) had loss of internal

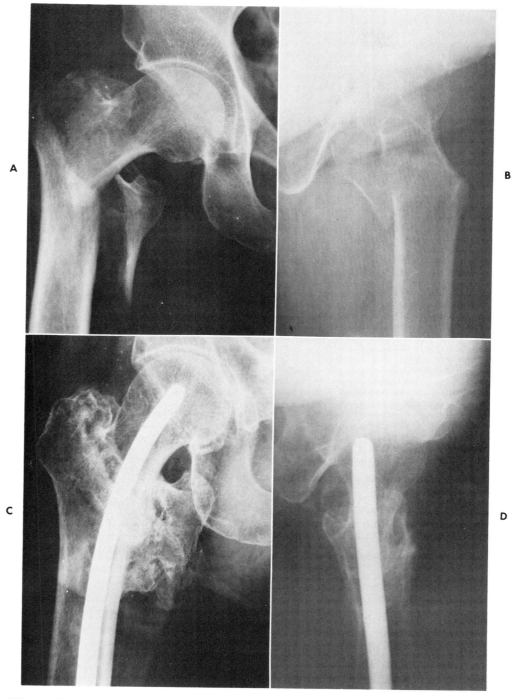

Fig. 2-10. A, Anteroposterior roentgenogram of an unstable intertrochanteric fracture in a 69-year-old woman with spastic hemiparesis. There is severe posterior comminution and a large, separate posteromedial fragment. **B,** Lateral roentgenogram demonstrates posterior comminution. Patient underwent closed nailing and began weight bearing 1 week postoperatively. **C** and **D,** Anteroposterior and lateral roentgenograms 1 year after surgery demonstrate fracture union.

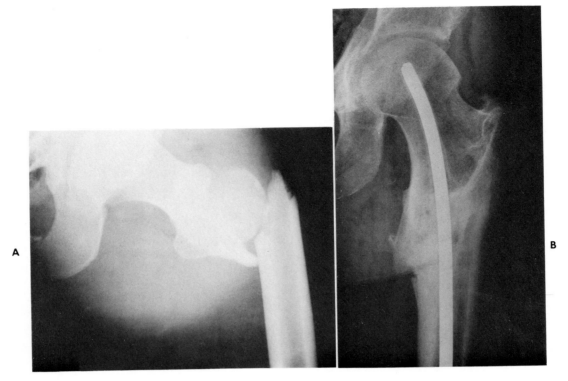

Fig. 2-11. A, Anteroposterior roentgenogram of a stable subtrochanteric fracture in a 33-year-old man. Following closed nailing, the patient began weight bearing at 1 week. **B,** Anteroposterior roentgenogram 1 year after surgery demonstrates fracture union.

rotation of 15 degrees or greater (15 to 35 degrees) when compared to the nonfractured hip. The external rotation deformities were evident immediately postoperatively and were, therefore, attributed to technical errors in obtaining accurate rotatory reductions. The incidence of this complication has been substantially reduced by careful attention to rotatory alignment at the time of surgery.

Varus deformity. Three intertrochanteric and two subtrochanteric fractures healed with varus deformities of 7 to 15 degrees. None of these five patients demonstrated limitation in range of motion of the hip or knee, and all regained full function. However, every effort should be made to avoid varus reductions at the time of surgery to minimize risks of loss of fracture fixation. (See discussion of complete loss of reduction.)

Knee pain. Most patients experienced some limitation in knee motion, which resolved during the first or second postoperative week. Four patients had persistent knee pain and limitation of motion related to protrusion of the distal end of the nail into the quadriceps mechanism. These nails were removed from 4 months to 1 year after the fracture, and a painless full range of knee motion ensued in each case. It should be noted that impaction at the fracture site is associated with relative distal displacement of the nail in the femoral shaft. Therefore, at surgery it is important to select a nail with a length that allows for its distal end to be countersunk at least 2 cm within the medullary canal.

Increased comminution of the fracture. In five patients (2.7%), further fragmentation at the fracture site was produced by the nailing procedure. In retrospect, nondisplaced fracture lines were often evident on preoperative roentgenograms. (The need for a careful inspection of preoperative roentgenograms cannot be overemphasized.) Postoperative ambulation was delayed 3 weeks in two of these patients, and all fracures united without further complication.

Comminution of the medial femoral cortex at the nail insertion site. Seven patients (3.8%) had comminution of the medial femoral condyle at

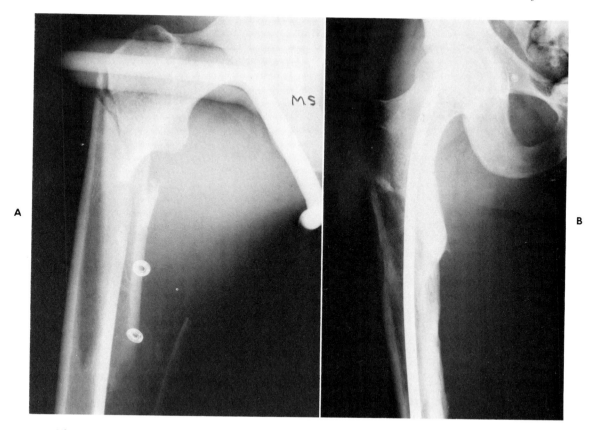

Fig. 2-12. A, Anteroposterior roentgenogram of an unstable subtrochanteric fracture in a 35-year-old man. There is a separate, large posteromedial fragment. Following closed nailing, the patient was treated in balanced suspension for 3½ weeks before weight bearing was allowed. **B,** Anteroposterior roentgenogram at 7½ months demonstrates fracture union.

the nail insertion site. This complication resulted from inserting the nail posterior to the femoral canal or levering the nail at the cortical window to manipulate the distal fragment. The thin cortical bone in the condylar region in elderly patients is relatively fragile and requires gentle surgical handling. Although this complication undoubtedly has contributed to postoperative knee pain, late knee function has not been affected.

Complete loss of reduction. Three unstable intertrochanteric fractures and one unstable subtrochanteric fracture had loss of fracture reduction (2.8%). Failures of fixation of the intertrochanteric fractures were associated with varus reduction in one case and placement of the nail insufficiently deep within the femoral head in another. The third intertrochanteric fracture lost reduction despite what appeared to be a technically sat-

isfactory nailing. The single unstable subtrochanteric fracture that lost reduction occurred in an 81-year-old man who had a relatively wide medullary canal and a long spiral fracture. In retrospect, supplemental fixation should have been used to safely allow early mobilization of this patient. Three of the four patients just cited underwent renailings with satisfactory results. When one takes into account the nails removed because of knee pain (four), there were seven secondary procedures required (3.8%).

Mortality. There were no surgical deaths. There were 8 deaths out of 216 patients (3.7%) during the first 6 postoperative weeks and a total of 17 deaths out of 202 patients (8.4%) followed up for at least 8 months. Holt, Ecker, and Sarmiento[4,10,17] report early postoperatively mortality rates of 12% to 16%. Nieman and Mankin reported a 6-week mortality rate of 36.5% in geriatric, institutionalized patients. In their series, after 6 weeks, the mortality rate was similar to institutionalized patients without fractures.[18] Miller found a 27% mortality rate of hip fracture patients at 1 year, compared to a 9% mortality of a comparable population without fractures. Mortality correlated with age of the patient and the presence of mental deterioration.[17] Jensen[12] reported a 1-year mortality rate of 26.8% and noted that survival rates had not improved over the previous 15 years. The mean patient age of 75 in this series is consistent with the mean ages of 73 to 81.6 reported in the series cited.* Factors, such as the incidence of cerebral dysfunction, cardiovascular disease, and other major medical complications, may vary significantly in different populations and account for variations in mortality rates. Nevertheless, the 8-month mortality rate of 8.4% in this series seems to represent a substantial improvement in patient survival. The improved survival rate can be attributed to reduced operative trauma, no infections, and earlier ambulation.

SUMMARY

Condylocephalic nailing of intertrochanteric and subtrochanteric fractures reduces operative time, surgical exposure, blood loss, and risks of postoperative infection compared to standard open hip nailing techniques. The nail is orientated approximately parallel to loading forces on the proximal femur and permits early weight-bearing in most cases. This procedure is relatively new, and many of the orthopaedic complications reported can be attributed to the learning process of defining technical pitfalls, indications, and contraindications. The mortality rate (8.4% at 8 months) and complications that are potentially life-threatening to these patients (2.7% fixation failures and 3.8% secondary procedures) are significantly lower than in other reported series of extracapsular hip fractures.† This technique, therefore, appears to be most advantageous for patients in poor health who are high operative risks.

Experience with condylocephalic nailing of subtrochanteric fractures has been limited. However, the fixation failure rate of only one out of

fifty-two fractures (2%) suggests that this technique offers a promising alternative to other implants designed for the fixation of subtrochanteric fractures.

REFERENCES

1. Bradley, G. W., et al.: The effects of mechanical environment on fracture healing, Orthop. Res. Soc. **2:**129, 1977.
2. Brown, S. A., Major, M. B., and Vandergraff, S.: The use of polyester materials for fracture fixation, Orthop. Res. Soc. **3:**3, 1978.
3. Cobey, J., et al.: Indicators of recovery from fractures of the hip, Clin. Orthop. **117:**258, 1976.
4. Counts, R., et al.: Comparison of stainless steel and composite plates in the healing of diaphyseal osteotomies of the dog radius, Ortho. Clin. **7:**223, 1976.
5. Dimon, J. H., and Hughston, J. C.: Unstable intertrochanteric fractures of the hip, J. Bone Joint Surg. **49-A:**440, April, 1967.
6. Ecker, M. C., Joyce, J. J., and Kohl, E. J.: The treatment of trochanteric hip fractures using a compression screw, J. Bone Joint Surg. **57-A:**23, Jan., 1975.
7. Evans, E. M.: The treatment of trochanteric fractures of the femur, J. Bone Joint Surg. **31-B:**190, May, 1949.
8. Herrero, F. C., Brichs, J. W., and Beltran, J. E.: Condylocephalic nail fixation for trochanteric fractures of the femur, Ortho. Clin. **5:**669, 1974.
9. Herrero, F. C., Villa, J., and Beltran, J. E.: Condylocephalic nail fixation for trochanteric fractures of the femur, J. Bone Joint Surg. **55-B:**774, Nov., 1973.
10. Holt, E. P.: Hip fractures in the trochanteric region: treatment with a strong nail and early weight bearing, J. Bone Joint Surg. **45-A:**687, June, 1963.
11. Inman, M. D.: Functional aspects of the abductor muscles of the hip, J. Bone Joint Surg. **29:**607, 1947.
12. Jensen, J. S., and Tondevold, E.: Mortality after hip fractures, Acta Orthop. Scand. **50:**161, 1979.
13. Kuderna, H., Bohler, N., and Collon, D.: Treatment of intertrochanteric and subtrochanteric fractures of the hip by the Ender method, J. Bone Joint Surg. **58-A:**604, July, 1976.
14. Kuntscher, G.: A new method of treatment of peritrochanteric fractures, Proc. R. Soc. Med. **63:**1120, Nov. 1970.
15. Lezius, A.: Intramedullary nailing of intertrochanteric and subtrochanteric fractures with curved nail, J. Int. Coll. Surg. **13:**569, May, 1950.
16. Massie, W. K.: Fractures of the hip, J. Bone Joint Surg. **46-A:**658, April, 1964.
17. Miller, C. W.: Survival and ambulation following hip fracture, J. Bone Joint Surg. **60-A:**930, 1978.
18. Nieman, K. M. W., and Mankin, H. J.: Fractures about the hip in an institutionalized patient population, J. Bone Joint Surg. **50-A:**1327, Oct., 1968.
19. Sarmiento, A.: Intertrochanteric fractures of the femur, J. Bone Joint Surg. **45-A:**706, June, 1963.
20. Seinsheimer, F.: Subtrochanteric fractures of the femur, J. Bone Joint Surg. **60-A:**300, April, 1978.
21. Spotoff, J.: Osteosynthesis of the neck of the femur, J. Bone Joint Surg **31-A:**836, 1949.

---

*See references 4, 10, 12, 17, and 18.
†See references 5, 6, 10, 16, and 19.

22. Swartz, A. D., Salamon, P. B., and Wigbe, D. A.: Treatment and mortality in intertrochanteric fractures of the hip—a graphic review, Ortho. Rev. **5**:47, June, 1976.
23. Uhthoff, H., and Dubuc, F.: Bone structure changes in the dog under rigid internal fixation, Clin. Orthop. **81**:165, 1971.
24. Watson, K., Campbell, R., and Wade, A.: Classification, treatment, and complications of the adult subtrochanteric fractures, J. Trauma **4**:457, 1964.
25. Woo, S., et al.: A comparison of cortical bone atrophy secondary to fixation with plates with large differences in bending stiffness, J. Bone Joint Surg. **50-A**:190, 1976.

Part II

Condylocephalic nailing of intertrochanteric fractures

DANA M. STREET

HISTORY

Nailing of intertrochanteric fractures of the femur from the medial side began with Lezius and Herzer[18] in 1951, who inserted the nail at the junction of the middle and proximal third of the femur. In 1964, Küntscher dropped the point of insertion to the medial condyle where the cortex is thinner and the thinner soft tissue requires less exposure. He first described condylocephalic nailing in the German literature in 1966[15,16] and again in English in 1970.[17] Collado, Mijiers, Beltran, and Vila[1,4] in Barcelona, Spain, reported their series in 1969, 1972, and 1973, following Küntscher's technique in all respects. This included the insertion of a guide pin in the region of the medial condyle after piercing the cortex and entering the medullary canal with an awl, then driving the pin up the medullary canal into the femoral neck and head, and rotating it as necessary to reduce the fracture. A prebent 10 mm cloverleaf nail was then driven over the guide pin, and the pin was removed. A flat pin was then driven through the eye in the distal end of the nail to prevent it from backing out (Fig. 2-13).

In 1970, Ender and Simon-Weidner[8,9,19] published the first accounts of nailing the intertrochanteric fracture using three pins that were smaller and more flexible and patterned after the $^3/_{16}$ inch Rush pin. They presented this as a further development of Küntscher's idea and reported a 1-year experience.

The point of insertion was moved more proximally to the flare of the condyle above the epicon-

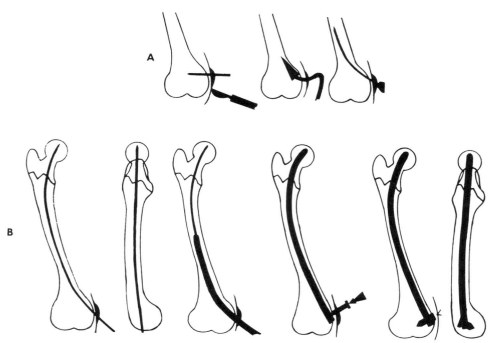

Fig. 2-13. Technique by Küntscher. **A,** Introduction of the guide pin. **B,** Introduction of the nails. (From Küntscher, G.: Proc. R. Soc. Med. **63**:1120, 1970.)

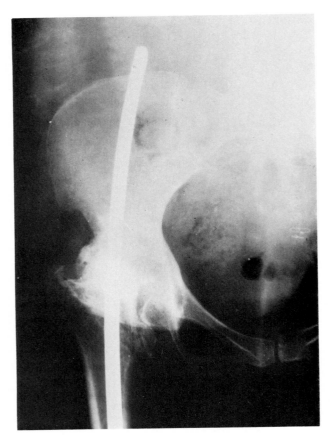

Fig. 2-14. Intertrochanteric fracture in patient with severe arthritis and restriction of hip motion. Nail traverses hip joint and wing of ilium in manner of Schneider hip fusion.

dyle, which interfered less with the knee joint. A subsequent report by Ender and Simon-Weidner[10] in 1974 shows modification of the hook end of the Rush pins to a flattened end with a hole, which allowed the use of a hook extractor, and the nails were prebent. This report also states that a fourth pin is sometimes necessary in large canals.

Among other papers by Ender's son,[6] also in German, is one illustrating reduction of the fracture by rotating the first pin. He also speaks of the need for a fourth and even a fifth nail in osteoporotic bones with wide canals. There has thus been a gradual recognition of the need for more nails to fill larger canals. Böhler[3] has used as many as ten nails in one case. A more recent paper in English by Kuderna, Böhler, and Collon[14] in 1976 gives an excellent account of the principles and technique of this method.

My experience with this method began in 1973, when, after reading Collado's report, I encountered an intertrochanteric fracture in an arthritic patient with minimal hip motion. I thought that the usual nailplates would fail because of the long lever of the lower extremity acting on the fracture site with an immobile hip joint. Therefore, an 11 mm Hansen-Street nail was inserted into the medial condyle and driven up the medullary canal and through the neck and head of the femur, across the hip joint, and up through the wing of the ilium in the manner of a Schneider hip fusion (Fig. 2-14). The patient, who was followed up for 5 months, progressed satisfactorily, then was lost to follow-up.

ANATOMY OF THE FEMUR

The femur bows anteriorly approximately 1 cm and somewhat less laterally over its entire length. The anterior surfaces of the condyles are approximately flush with the anterior surface of the shaft, and the diameter of the condyles is more than twice that of the midshaft. Therefore, the medial epicondyle near the center of the condyle is considerably posterior to the medullary canal of the shaft. The neck of the femur has a forward angulation, or anteversion, which, according to Gray,[2] "is extremely variable, but on an average is from 21 to 14 degrees." According to Dunlap et al.,[5] it averages 8.70 degrees. We have found it may also differ in the femurs of the same individual (Fig. 2-15). Kingsley and Olmsted[13] found a range from minus 20 degrees minimum to plus 38 degrees maximum with a similar average of 8.02 degrees in a series of 630 adult femurs. Interestingly, the right femur averaged about 1 degree more than the left.

DESIGN OF NAILS

Since the nail must enter the femur medial to the shaft, traverse the medullary canal, and curve again medially into the neck and femoral head, the basic curve of the nail is a bow of approximately 4 to 5 cm from a straight line, most of which is in the proximal and distal thirds. A nail inserted at the medial epicondyle must curve anteriorly to get into the medullary canal. It then continues to bow anteriorly in the anterior bow of the shaft, and, if the nail has a flat curve in a single plane, it then bows posteriorly in the proximal end. If the fracture has been reduced and the external rotation corrected, the nail will ei-

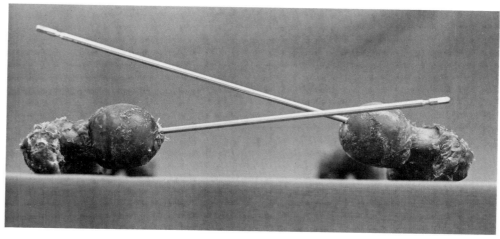

Fig. 2-15. Angle of anteversion in femurs from same individual. Right measures 6 degrees; left measures 2 degrees.

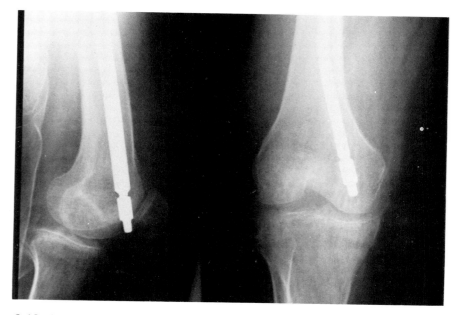

Fig. 2-16. Anteroposterior and lateral views showing point of insertion close to knee joint and midway between patella and medial epicondyle.

ther lodge too far posteriorly in the neck and head or pass posterior to the neck altogether. This can be avoided by bending the nail anteriorly in the proximal 5 to 10 cm of nail length. A 7- to 10-degree anteversion angle is probably about right for a prebent nail, but one should be able to increase or decrease the bend as the situation may require.

In my first 46 cases, in which a single 11 mm Hansen-Street nail was used, the nail was inserted more anteriorly midway between the medial epicondyle and the medial margin of the patella and just proximal to the knee joint (Fig. 2-16). This allowed the nail to bow more laterally in the shaft and correspondingly medially rather than posteriorly at the neck and head. The curve

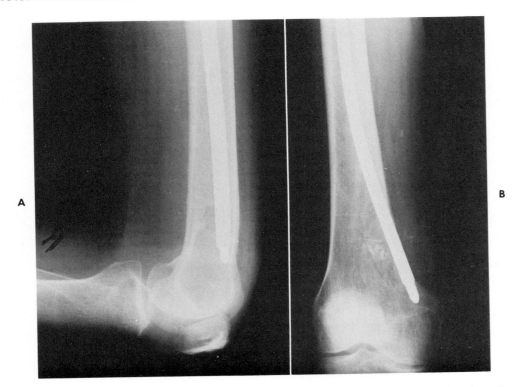

Fig. 2-17. A, Lateral view. **B,** Anteroposterior view showing more proximal point of insertion on flare of condyle interfering less with knee function. Comminution of cortex proximal to window presents no problem.

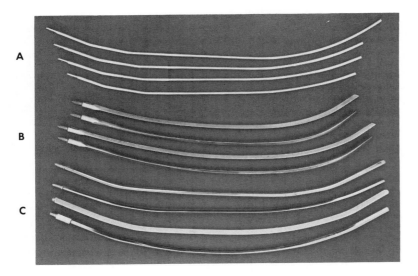

Fig. 2-18. A, Four Ender nails. **B,** Harris nails. **C,** Hansen-Street nails. Ender and Harris nails come prebowed. Hansen-Street nails come straight and are bowed at the operating table. Lower three nails in **A** and **C** were removed from patients.

of the nail thrusting against the lateral cortex also added to the stability of the nail in the medullary canal with less tendency for the nail to back out and oblique fragments to override. We attempted to drive the nail to the point where the threaded stud hung against the cortex. There was very little leeway. If the nail projected too far medially, was even 1 cm too long, or backed out 1 cm, it would interfere with the gliding of the retinaculum with knee motion and cause pain even though it did not impinge against the tibia.

Because the nail interfered with the knee joint, we have since moved our point of insertion to a more proximal position at the flare of the condyle, as recommended by Ender (Fig. 2-17). This, again, is more in line with the medullary canal and allows the nail to bow laterally. The only modification in nail design is that it bows less in the distal than proximal end, since it does not have to project so far medially. This is also true of the Ender and Harris nails (Fig. 2-18).

Some have recommended that the nail have three components to its curve, that is, to angle anteriorly at the proximal end for the anteversion, bow anteriorly over its entire length for the anterior bow of the medullary canal, and curve medially and posteriorly at the distal end to bring it out through the condyle. This twist, or corkscrew curve, more nearly fits the inside of the femur. It drives in easily, but it also backs out with equal ease. A nail with a flat curve directed laterally is much more stable.

MECHANICAL PROPERTIES OF NAILS

Two factors were investigated regarding the mechanical characteristics of the Ender, Harris, and Hansen-Street nails: the bending or yield strength and the elasticity or springiness. Bending strength was measured directly by clamping the nail in a vise and hanging weights at a measured distance from the vise. The deflection was then recorded on paper behind the nail by drawing along its upper surface as increments of weight were added. The weight was released after each increase, and the base line was again drawn to make sure the nail had sprung back to its original position and had not slipped in the vise. Weights were added until an amount was reached that produced a permanent deformation (Fig. 2-19). The amount of deflection before deformation was considered a function of elasticity, and the maximum was noted for the different nails. The min-

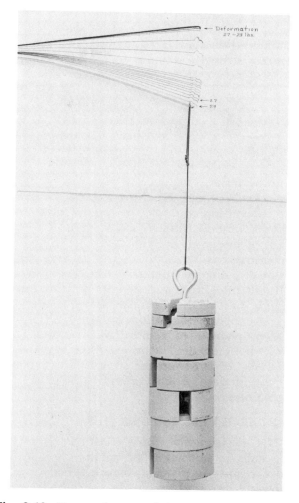

Fig. 2-19. Hansen-Street nail loaded with 5 lb increments (up to 20 lb) returned to the original line each time when unloaded. Weight was then increased by 1 lb amounts. Deformation began at 28 lb. Moment arm is 37.6 cm.

imum weight required to produce a permanent deformation was considered the bending or yield strength.

The Ender nails, being of considerably less diameter, supported less weight than the Hansen-Street or Harris nails and, therefore, had lower yield strength. It required six Ender nails to equal one 11 by 8 mm Hansen-Street nail in bending strength, even though the former have a combined cross-sectional area of 95 sq mm, while the latter is only 44 sq mm. Again, this would be expected, since a solid cable is stiffer than a stranded cable. The amount of deflection for each increment and total weight (i.e., the elasticity) was the same for the Hansen-Street nail and Ender nails (3% variation), both being No. 316 stainless steel. The Harris titanium nail showed a bending strength identical to the Hansen-Street stainless steel nail; however, elasticity was 21.6% greater.

In using the diamond-shaped Hansen-Street nail in this method, we have started with the straight 11 mm nail and bent it at the operating table using two 15-inch (38 cm) lengths of pipe as benders, which scar the nail less than the usual bending irons. This has two advantages over using a prebent nail. First, the nail can be bent to the anteversion angle needed proximally and the amount of bow distally, which depends on the point of insertion. Secondly, we have found that nails vary considerably in their elasticity, and, occasionally, one encounters a nail that is far too soft and straightens out when driven through the straight part of the medullary canal. It then fails to curve medially again into the neck and head. It is then possible to remove the nail and "cold work" it by bending it an excessive amount, for example, 15 cm from the straight line and back to the desired 5 cm, thereby increasing the springiness.

ELECTROLYTIC PROPERTIES OF NAILS

The electromotive force (EMF) developed by two nails in normal saline solution was investigated relative to possible corrosion, bone lysis, or deposition around an anode or cathode where multiple nails are used, as in the Ender technique, and where combinations of different nails are used. A direct measurement of current was made with a simple apparatus, which immersed the nails to a standard depth of 10 cm for easy calculation of surface area. They were a measured distance apart and connected to a microammeter through a key.

There was found to be a sudden flow of current reaching a peak and falling again in a few seconds to approximately one tenth of the peak amount, where it remained fairly constant. This rapid drop was attributed to polarization, and the lesser current was thought to represent the usual state in the body. Averages of multiple tests with the same nails, different nails from the same manufacture, nails of the same alloy from different manufacturers, and nails made of different alloys (i.e., Harris' titanium nail vs. stainless steel) was determined. It was soon found that there

were gross discrepancies between the initial test and subsequent tests, even though such factors as a possible static charge on the nails, capacitive charge, and a possible surface coating from polarization were eliminated. The initial test was consistently greater and was used as a basis for comparison.

A considerable variation in nails of the same type and manufacture was found. Ender nails showed an initial peak ranging from 3 to 30 μA or 3 μA sustained. One might suspect the greater amount might cause some corrosion over a period of years and might be a reason for removing the nails once the fracture is solidly united. Rush nails and Hansen-Street nails, by different manufacturers, gave slightly higher readings when tested with Ender nails, but when corrected for surface area were in the same range. Harris vs stainless steel nails gave no higher readings than the maximum readings of stainless steel vs stainless steel nails.

The EMF of different combinations of nails was also tested with a high resistance circuit by using an oscilloscope, and, again, they showed a wide range of 3 to 300 mV (average 96 mV). Unlike during the current determinations, the surface area immersed made no difference. Static charges caused a considerable effect. In the low resistance (current) tests, the high initial reading dropped in a few seconds to one tenth of the initial reading. The potential dropped immediately when short circuited, that is, converted to low resistance. Again, the drop in potential was attributed to polarization. The low resistance tests are thought to more nearly parallel the situation in the body where nails are in contact.

CLINICAL EXPERIENCES WITH HANSEN-STREET NAILS

It was my initial contention that a nail could be driven anywhere that a guide pin could be driven; thus a Hansen-Street nail could be used instead of a guide pin and Küentscher nail. In general, this has proven true, particularly when the fracture is in satisfactory position at the time the nail is driven, as in an undisplaced fracture, a reduced fracture, or a fracture to be nailed in unreduced position. The diamond nail does not rotate readily in the medullary canal as does a guide pin or Ender nail. This has both disadvantages and advantages. It cannot be inserted into the neck and rotated to help reduce the fracture,

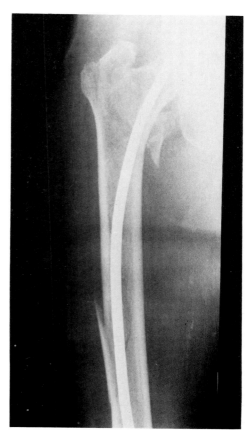

Fig. 2-20. Fracture in lateral cortex of shaft incurred when nail was driven. There is some loss of stability in shaft. There were no problems in healing or removing nail.

but it is more stable once in position. It has, therefore, proven an excellent fixator for the relatively undisplaced fracture in the elderly patient who would heal without any treatment if he could be kept off it, but is likely to bear weight and displace it. Also, it is inserted more quickly than multiple nails in these poor surgical risk patients.

The strong lateral pressure of the single diamond nail may lead to the complication of fracturing the lateral cortex when the nail is driven (Fig. 2-20) in the severely osteoporotic patient. This occurred three times in 55 cases. Although only the lateral cortex was involved and it healed with no problem, this situation would be an indication for using multiple Ender nails, since each nail would exert much less lateral thrust while inserting. In no case was the medial cortex penetrated by the nail.

Although most physicians use a fracture table

for these patients, we have found an ordinary operating table to be satisfactory. The fracture is usually easily reduced by manual traction and internal rotation, and when the extremity is draped free, it is more easily manipulated. If a biplane image intensifier is used, a fracture table might be preferable. However, having only one image intensifier (which is a must for this procedure), we leave it in the anteroposterior (AP) position and flex the hip to 90 degrees (frog leg) for the lateral view, rather than shifting the image intensifier back and forth between AP and lateral positions, which is often required. Many x-ray technicians are not very adept at making the change.

CLINICAL EXPERIENCES WITH ENDER NAILS

Ender nails have been advocated for treatment of subtrochanteric fractures[2,7] and combined intertrochanteric and shaft fractures. For the subtrochanteric fracture, my preference has been a straight nail, supplemented with screws for comminution as necessary[11] (Fig. 2-21), which avoids possible complications at the hip joint. In combined intertrochanteric and shaft fractures there is a tendency toward a lateral bow of the shaft with condylocephalic nailing unless the central part of the nail is made straighter. It then loses some of its fixation in the canal that is gained by springing against the lateral cortex. The lateral bow can be counteracted by inserting Ender nails in the lateral condyle and curving them up into the greater trochanter.[2,7]

We, too, have run into the need for more than three Ender nails when the vertical fracture line tends toward overriding and instability. A patient with three nails (Fig. 2-22, *A*) showed 2 cm overriding 1 month later (Fig. 2-22, *B*). One nail became trapped inside the cortex at the distal end and penetrated the head, involving the hip joint. The other two pins were pushed distally. It was necessary to reduce the fracture again, reposition the three nails, and insert two more Ender nails, after which the patient's convalescence was uneventful (Fig. 2-22, *C*).

A patient with an unstable four-part fracture was satisfactorily fixated with four Ender nails plus one Rush nail (Fig. 2-23) inserted from above through the lateral trochanteric fragment. These pins were removed at 7 months and showed no evidence of corrosion.

The Ender nails with divergence in the femoral

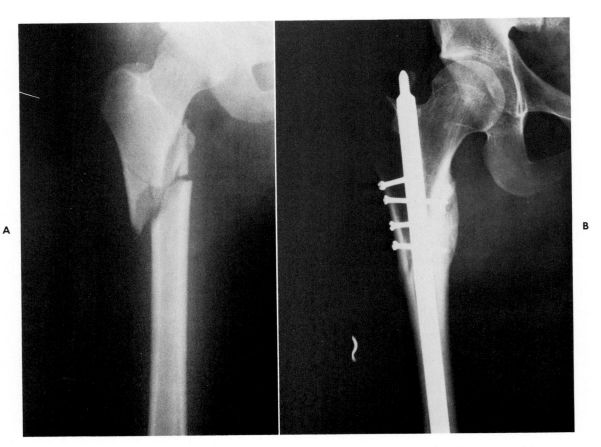

Fig. 2-21. A, Comminuted subtrochanteric fracture. **B,** Fracture optimally treated with straight nail and supplementary screws.

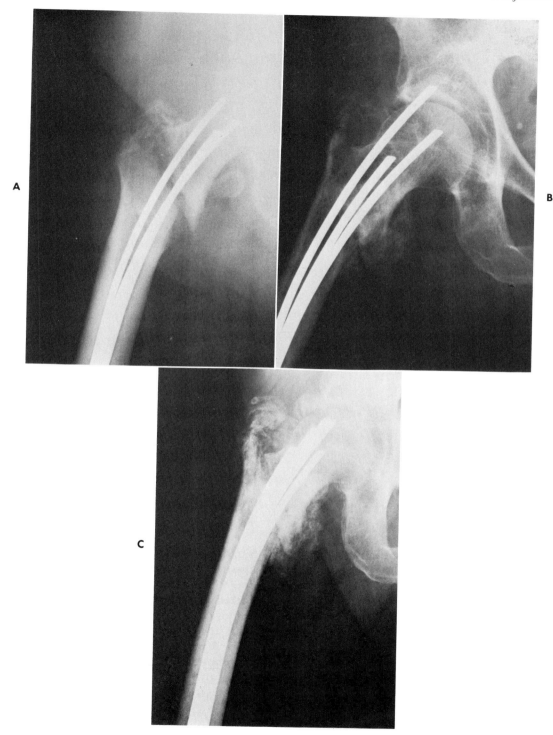

Fig. 2-22. A, Intertrochanteric fracture initially treated with three Ender nails. **B,** At 1 month they had overridden 2 cm. One nail trapped distally was pushed into the hip joint, while the other two backed out. **C,** The fracture was again reduced; the nails were re-positioned, and two more Ender nails were inserted, after which the fracture remained stable.

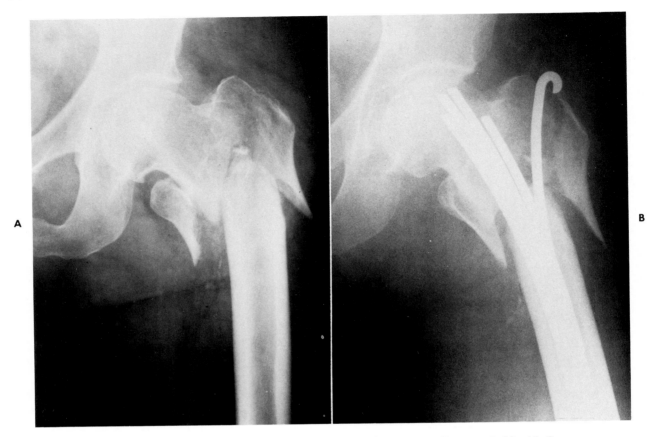

Fig. 2-23. A, Unstable four-part intertrochanteric fracture. **B,** Fracture held with four Ender nails plus one Rush nail in the lateral trochanteric fragment. The nails showed no corrosion when removed at 7 months.

head secure a better hold on the head to control torque and angulation than a single nail in the center of the head.[2] A single large nail, on the other hand, has the advantage of more stable fixation in the medullary canal. A combination of the two types of nails might, therefore, be more stable than either type alone. We have placed two Ender nails in the anterior and posterior of the head and a Hansen-Street nail between them (Fig. 2-24). This combination provided the equivalent of eight Ender nails in terms of resistance to bending. In two patients, the Hansen-Street nail, plus the two Ender nails, filled the canal snugly. In another patient, in whom this combination was inserted with little resistance, a third Ender nail was added with difficulty.

SUMMARY

Condylocephalic nailing was developed by Küntscher in 1964 as an extension of the medial intramedullary nailing of Lezius. This method was further developed by Ender and Simon-Weidner in 1969 with the use of multiple, more slender, elastic nails. My own experience with this method, commencing in 1973, made use of the solid diamond-shaped Hansen-Street nail inserted just above the anteromedial margin of the femoral joint surface. Because of disturbances with the knee joint, the point of insertion was moved more proximally to the condylar flare, as recommended by Ender. Resistance to bending stress of the Hansen-Street and Harris nails was found to be about equal to six Ender nails. The current developed and the potential differences were found to vary considerably between stainless steel nails by the same manufacturer, stainless steel nails by different manufacturers, and between stainless steel and titanium alloy nails. However, they were all in the same general range of 3 to 30 μA and 3 to 300 mV. More than three

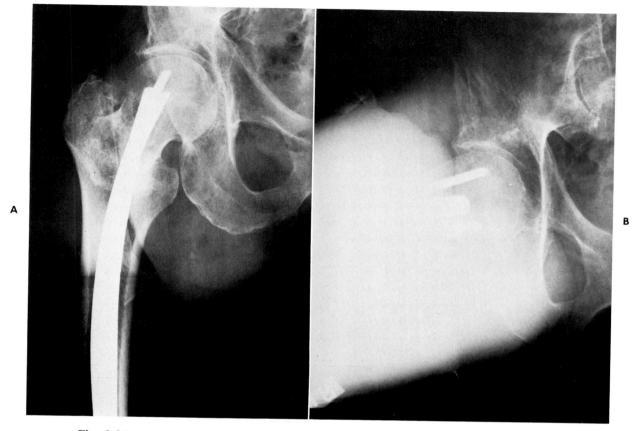

Fig. 2-24. A, Intertrochanteric fracture firmly fixed with one Hansen-Street nail and two Ender nails. **B,** Lateral view shows location of Ender nails in anterior and posterior of head with diamond nail in the center.

Ender nails are frequently needed, and fixation is improved by filling the canal. Fixation in both the femoral head and medullary canal may be improved by a combination of nails, such as one Hansen-Street and two Ender nails.

REFERENCES

1. Beltran, J. E.: Condylocephalic nail in pertrochanteric fractures of the neck of the femur, J. Bone Joint Surg. **54-B:**748, 1972.
2. Böhler, J.: In The hip, vol. 3, St. Louis, 1975, The C. V. Mosby Co.
3. Böhler, J.: The Spectator, July 10, 1978.
4. Collado, F., Vila, J., and Beltran, J. E.: Condylocephalic nail fixation for trochanteric fractures of the femur, J. Bone Joint Surg. **55-B:**774, 1973.
5. Dunlap, K., Shands, A. R., Jr., Hollister, L. C., Jr., Gaul, J. S., Jr., and Streit, H. W.: A new method for determination of torsion of the femur, J. Bone Joint Surg. **35-A:**289, 1953.
6. Ender, H. G.: Fixierung trochanterer Frakturen mit elastichen Kondylennägeln, Chir. Praxis **18:**81, 1974.
7. Ender, H. G., and Schneider, H.: Subtrochantere Brüche des Oberschenkels: Berhandlung mit Fedenagela, Aktuel. Chir. **9:**359, 1974.
8. Ender, J.: Probleme beim frischen per- und subtrochanteren Oberschenkelbruch, Hefte Unfallheilkd **106:**2, 1970.
9. Ender, J., and Simon-Weidner, R.: Die Fixierung der trochanteren Brüche mit runden elastischen Condylennägeln, Acta Chir. Austriaca **1:**40, 1970.
10. Ender, J., and Simon-Weidner, R.: Die Fixierung der Brüche des Trochantermassivs mit elastischen Rundnägeln, Aktuel. Chir. **9:**71, 1974.
11. Funk, F. J., Jr., Wells, R. E., and Street, D. M.: Supplementary fixation of femoral fractures, Clin. Orthop. **60:**41, 1968.
12. Gray, H.: Anatomy of the human body, ed. 22, Philadelphia, 1930, Lea & Febiger.
13. Kingsley, P. C., and Olmsted, K. L.: A study to determine the angle of anteversion of the neck of the femur, J. Bone Joint Surg. **30-A:**745, 1948.
14. Kuderna, H., Böhler, N., and Collon, D. J.: Treatment of intertrochanteric and subtrochanteric fractures of the hip by the Ender method, J. Bone Joint Surg. **58-A:**604, 1976.

15. Küntscher, G.: Zur operativen Behandlung der pertrochanteren Fraktur, Zentralbl. Chir. **9:**281, 1966.

16. Küntscher, G.: Weitere Fortschritte auf dem gebiet der Marknagelung, Langenbecks Arch. Chir. **316:**224, 1966.

17. Küntscher, G.: A new method of treatment of pertrochanteric fractures, Proc. R. Soc. Med. **63:**1120, 1970.

18. Lezius, A.: Intramedullary nailing of intertrochanteric and subtrochanteric fractures, J. Int. Coll. Surg. **13:**569, 1950.

19. Simon-Weidner, R.: Die Fixierung trochanterer Brüche mit multiplen elastischen Rundnägeln nach Simon-Weidner, Hefte Unfallheilkd. **106:**60, 1970.

Chapter 3

The A.O. (ASIF)* method of fracture care

JOSEPH SCHATZKER

MARVIN TILE

It is the purpose of this chapter to introduce our philosophy of fracture care. It is based on the A.O.† method of internal fixation, but we have adapted it to a North American practice. The A.O. was founded in 1958 by several Swiss surgeons unhappy with the methods of internal fixation available to them at that time. Since both authors were in residency training during that same period, we agree that methods of internal fixation of fractures at that period left much to be desired. The Swiss surgeons embarked on a most ambitious task, which was to assess the then current methods of treatment and to see if those methods could be improved. This was done by careful documentation of fracture cases and critical analysis of each case. It eventually led to the evolution of new principles, new methods, and new implants, which we shall discuss in this chapter.

We shall not advocate internal fixation of all fractures as some would believe but will stress that many fractures can and should be managed conservatively. The major contribution of A.O. to fracture care has been in the evolution of new principles and techniques of internal fixation, not in surgical judgment. The astute clinician, therefore, will use clinical judgment to determine the most suitable methods of fracture care for patients. If internal fixation is chosen for a fracture, we would then strongly recommend the adoption of the principles and techniques of the A.O. and not just the use of A.O. implants. There is little excuse for the inadequate internal fixation that one commonly encounters (Fig. 3-1), which gives

the worst of both worlds: inadequate internal fixation and consequent prolonged immobilization leading to delayed rehabilitation and permanent stiffness of the joints. Instead, we advocate such stable internal fixation that early motion of the limb without the need for external splintage is possible.

AIMS AND PRINCIPLES

The main aim in fracture care is the early return of the injured extremity to full function. It is evident that this statement does not imply a method of treatment, be it open or closed. In fact, the entire thrust in North America has been to achieve early return to full function by closed means, such as by early weight bearing and functional bracing of fractures. We agree with this and use these methods extensively in our fracture clinics. However, not all fractures should be treated by closed means. We feel that the indications for open reduction that will be discussed in detail later in this chapter include the following:

1. Intra-articular fractures (where technically possible)
2. Metaphyseal fractures, particularly in the lower extremity when associated with displacement and crush
3. Select diaphyseal fractures, especially forearm fractures
4. Complications of fractures, including nonunion and malunion
5. Miscellaneous indications, including multiple injuries, limb reimplantations, and major soft tissue and neurovascular injuries

Each fracture must be carefully studied, and the method of treatment chosen that will return

---

*Association for the Study of Internal Fixation.
†Arbeitsgemeindschaft für Osteosynthesefragen.

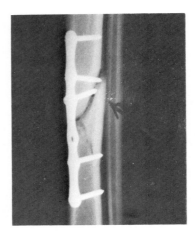

Fig. 3-1. Compression was not used to increase stability of internal fixation. Instead of being a lag screw, the third screw from the top is in the fracture line, as is the second; both block reduction. The main fragments are held apart by the plate, which is also too short.

the limb to full function as quickly as possible. The closed methods of functional bracing and weight-bearing plasters allow early rehabilitation and attempt to eliminate "fracture disease" by stable external means and early function. The A.O. open method of internal fixation attempts to eliminate "fracture disease" by such stable internal fixation that early motion and function is possible because prolonged postoperative plaster fixation is no longer necessary. We do not believe that the swelling and stiffness of joints associated with "fracture disease" in all patients are necessarily the result of immobilization in plaster. Some are associated with so-called sympathetic reflex dystrophies and do occasionally occur in a patient treated by open means. The "fracture disease" is the result of pain, immobilization, and loss of function.

METHOD

If internal fixation is the treatment of choice, early return to full function depends on the attainment of absolutely stable fixation of the fracture. It renders the fracture painless and permits full motion of the limb without external splints or plaster. This also implies that the bone is sufficiently strong to hold the implant and that the implant is sufficiently strong to maintain reduction long enough for union to occur. In joint fractures, especially of weight-bearing joints, open reduction should be anatomic for permanent re-

turn of full function. The surgery must be atraumatic in order to preserve blood supply to soft tissues and maintain the viability of the bony fragments. Each internal fixation is a race between bone union and implant failure. The more extensive the bone necrosis, the longer the time to union and the more likely the failure of the implant.

Stable internal fixation may be achieved by either compression or splintage. Compression is the best means of achieving absolutely stable fixation. Splintage (e.g., intramedullary nailing) restores structural stability to bone by splinting it, but as a method of fixation it is almost never absolutely stable.

Compression

Compression was investigated and used clinically by surgeons prior to the founding of the A.O. Key[3] and Charnley[1] demonstrated the use of the compression method. Danis[2] was first to demonstrate radiologically that diaphyseal fractures, when rigidly fixed under compression, healed without resorption and without radiologically demonstrable callus. Danis termed this phenomenon *primary* or *vascular bone union*.

The founders of A.O. attempted to determine the following:
1. Response of bone to compression
2. Duration that compression can be maintained
3. Meaning of primary bone union

Wagner[8] demonstrated that when compression was correctly applied, it did not lead to bone necrosis, but that bone responded to the increased load by remodeling, by hypertrophy of the haversian systems, and by reorientation of the newly laid down bone according to Wolff's law.

Perren[5] in a series of experiments using strain gauge instrumented plates demonstrated that compression in bone was usually maintained until union was complete. Intact and osteotomized living cortex under axial compression showed an identical curve of a sharp initial drop followed by a gradual decline toward zero over the next 3 to 4 months (Fig. 3-2). He showed that the initial drop was due to the viscoelastic property of bone and that the gradual decline was due to haversian remodeling. The fact that both curves remained the same indicated that with maintenance of rigid fixation, net resorption of necrotic bone ends adjacent to the fracture did not occur, allowing

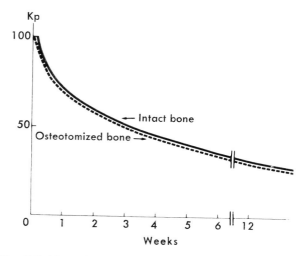

Fig. 3-2. Note that the rate of decay of compression in the intact and osteotomized bone is identical. During primary bone union, there is no net resorption at the fracture.

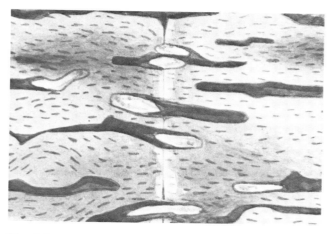

Fig. 3-3. Note the new haversian canals that are bridging the osteotomy. (From Müller, M. E., Allgower, M., and Willenegger, H.: Manual of internal fixation, New York, 1970, Springer-Verlag Publishing Co.)

compression to be sustained for at least as long as the experimental osteotomy needed to unite. A loss of 10 μm in substance at the fracture line would result in the sudden and total loss of compression. Therefore, the gradual decline meant that net resorption of the fracture zone never occurred as long as fixation remained stable. Resorption, as demonstrated in other experiments, is the result of motion.[6]

Schenk[7] studied the phenomenon of cortical bone healing under conditions of stable fixation. He was able to demonstrate that a bone stably fixed did in fact heal by primary bone formation across the fracture (Fig. 3-3). In areas of contact this union was accomplished by the development of new osteons, which bridged the fracture. Any bone resorbed was simultaneously replaced by osteoblasts that surrounded and advanced together with the new proliferating capillaries. Areas of gaps between bone healed first by woven bone, which was then gradually remodeled to lamellar bone by the development of new haversian systems.

Compression has no magic osteogenic properties, but it is the best method of securing stable fixation. We would stress, however, that primary bone union does not imply better bone union. The presence or absence of callus depends, of course, on many other factors. However, if a fracture has been stably fixed with a plate, the ap-

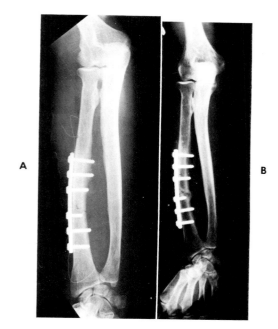

Fig. 3-4. A, Note gap in cortex opposite plate. **B,** At 6 weeks, the appearance of fluffy irregular "irritation callus," which is a sign of instability.

pearance of callus often signifies instability (Fig. 3-4). This type of callus is called *irritation callus.* It is not a favorable sign, for it signifies loss of fixation, movement of the fracture, and impending failure.

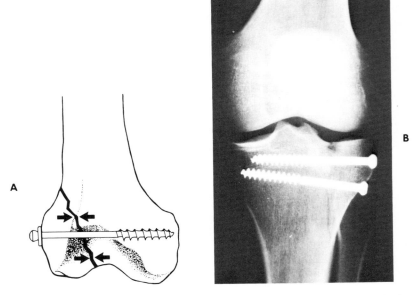

Fig. 3-5. A, The lag screw is the most basic and important method of achieving interfragmental compression. The thread must not cross fracture line. **B,** A.O. cancellous screws were used to lag together a Type I wedge–tibia-plateau fracture.

Compression may be achieved by the following means:

1. Interfragmental compression using the lag screw principle
2. Axial compression by tension band wiring, compression plates with tension device, self-compressing plates, such as dynamic compression plates (DCP) and semitabular plates, and external fixators
3. Combined methods of interfragmental and axial compression using neutralization and buttress plates

INTERFRAGMENTAL COMPRESSION

The lag screw is the most basic and important method of achieving interfragmental compression (Fig. 3-5, *A*). It is commonly used in the stabilization of intra-articular fractures, metaphyseal fractures, and diaphyseal fractures where the fracture line is at least twice as long as the diameter of the bone. The lag screw is the building block of stable internal fixation, and it is used in every instance where two loose fragments of bone can be compressed together even if the overall fixation will require other means, such as a neutralization plate, a buttress plate, or even an intramedullary nail.

The A.O. cancellous screw (Fig. 3-5, *B*) has been a great advance in fracture management. It is used in the treatment of fractures of the metaphysis and in joint fractures. A word of caution, however, to anyone attempting to fix extremely osteoporotic bone with these screws. Many metaphyseal fractures occur in elderly osteoporotic patients whose bone is not strong enough to hold the screw. Exacting techniques are important in this type of individual. A cancellous tap is not recommended in osteoporotic bone except to cut through the cortex under the screw head. Occasionally, if fixation of the screw fails, embedding it in cement will solve this difficult problem (Fig. 3-6).

The cortical screw is used as a lag screw by overdrilling the proximal cortex. If this is not done, the screw will maintain or keep the fracture apart as shown in Fig. 3-7. Cancellous screws are not used in diaphyseal regions as lag screws because with time bone fills the gliding hole right up to the shaft of the screw. At the time of screw removal the cancellous screw cannot cut a thread through cortex and often shears because of the excessive torque. The ingrowth of bone around the thread of a cortex screw does not hinder its removal.

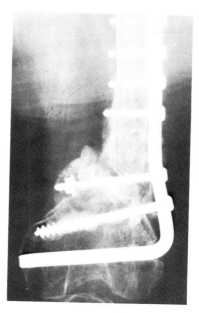

Fig. 3-6. Note cement plug surrounding the thread of the cancellous screw. Note also the nut used on the cortical screw just above. It is another method of improving the holding power of a screw in osteoporotic bone.

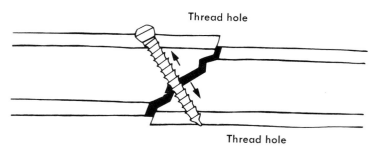

Fig. 3-7. Both holes are thread holes. The fragments will never come together. In order for this screw to compress the fragments, the hole in the cortex next to one screw head must be overdrilled. It will then become the "gliding hole."

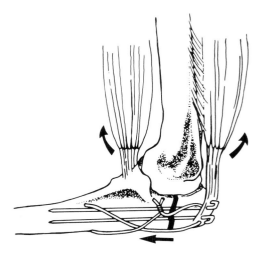

Fig. 3-8. Tension band wire fixation of the olecranon.

AXIAL COMPRESSION

Axial compression may be achieved by the following means:

1. Tension band wiring
2. Compression plates with tension devices
3. Self-compressing plates (DCP, semitubular plates)
4. External fixation

Tension band wire. Fractures at sites of tendinous or ligamentous attachments, such as fractures of the patella, olecranon, medial malleolus, greater trochanter, and occasionally of the greater and lesser tuberosity, can be stabilized by means of a tension band wire that neutralizes the distracting forces and brings the fracture under axial compression (Fig. 3-8). This principle of internal fixation is best illustrated in the schematic drawing of Pauwels (Fig. 3-9). It also finds application in certain bones such as the femur, which are eccentrically loaded. This results in one side of the bone being under tension and the other side under compression (Fig. 3-10). If fractured, such a bone can be stabilized by means of the tension band principle (Fig. 3-11), which leads to stable fixation of the fracture by means of axial compression.

Tension band plate. The tension device became the hallmark of A.O. (Fig. 3-11). It was developed as a means of setting either straight or angled blade plates under tension. These plates, once prestressed, are referred to as *tension band plates* (compression plates). They find their application in the treatment of eccentrically loaded bones such as the forearm, femur, humerus, and occasionally the tibia (especially in tibial nonunion).

There have been a number of excellent A.O. plates developed for almost all clinical situations. These plates may be used as tension band plates and neutralization or buttress plates. The terms tension band, neutralization, and buttress do not refer to the plate itself, but to the use to which it is put.

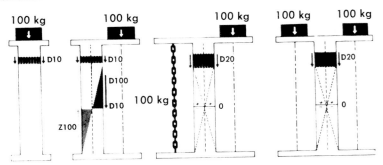

Fig. 3-9. Pauwels' schematic representation of the tension band principle. The chain represents the tension band. (From Müller, M. E., Allgower, M., and Willenegger, H.: Manual of internal fixation, New York, 1970, Springer-Verlag Publishing Co.)

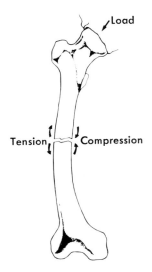

Fig. 3-10. When a load is applied eccentrically to a long bone, one cortex is loaded in compression and the other in tension.

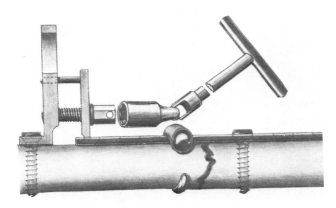

Fig. 3-11. The tension device. (From Müller, M. E., Allgower, M., and Willenegger, H.: Manual of internal fixation, New York, 1970, Springer-Verlag Publishing Co.)

Neutralization plate. The neutralization plate is essential in those clinical situations where interfragmental lag screw fixation alone is inadequate to overcome the sheer and torsional stresses acting upon the fracture. In comminuted fractures, fixation is secured by means of lag screws. A plate is then applied in such a way that it bridges the zone of comminution and conducts all forces from proximal to distal fragments bypassing the fracture (Fig. 3-12).

In comminuted fractures and in those fractures where bone loss has occurred, we strongly advocate the use of autogenous corticocancellous or cancellous bone grafts. In situations of comminution or bone loss, stability of the fixation often depends entirely on the holding power of the screws and the strength of the implant. Under these circumstances the bone is unable to withstand any stress because of its structural disruption. If bone is grafted by 6 to 8 weeks such fracture zones become bridged by an osteoid and osseous mass. Although still very weak, this mass is sufficiently strong to take part in stress transmission and in this way protect the internal fixation and the fixation of the fracture.

Buttress plate. In metaphyseal regions, where comminution of the cortex has occurred or where the cortex is so porotic as to be unable to withstand axial thrust, screw fixation should be supplemented by the use of a buttress plate. This

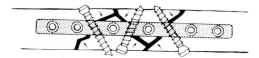

Fig. 3-12. Neutralization plate. A neutralization plate is fixed to the main fragments. It bridges the zone of communication and protects the lag screw fixation.

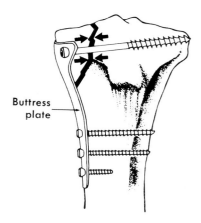

Fig. 3-13. The buttress plate supports the cortex and prevents displacement due to axial thrust.

plate supports the cortex and prevents slow progressive displacement of the fragments (Fig. 3-13). Its major application is in the treatment of intra-articular fractures and metaphyseal fractures of the proximal and distal tibia.

We do not recommend double plate fixation in diaphyseal fractures because of excessive stress protection and resultant porosis of the bone. However, double plates are occasionally necessary in metaphyseal fractures where they may be the only means of securing rigid fixation to allow early motion.

External skeletal fixation. Axial compression by means of external skeletal fixators has a limited role in the A.O. armamentarium. It is used largely in carrying out arthrodeses of the knee and ankle and in the treatment of certain metaphyseal nonunions. The external fixators, particularly the newly developed A.O. external fixator (tubular) and the Wagner leg lengthening apparatus, are much superior to the older types of external skeletal fixators. They are finding an ever greater application in the treatment of open fractures with major soft tissue damage and in the treatment of infected nonunions.

Splintage

INTRAMEDULLARY NAILING

The A.O. group claims no originality for this method and uses the principles elicited by Gerhard Kuentscher, that is, careful reaming of the medullary canal to obtain stable internal fixation by intramedullary splintage. Reaming allows the use of an adequate-sized nail sufficiently strong to overcome the forces of bending, rotation, and compression without external splintage. Intramedullary nail is the method of choice for internal fixation of transverse or short oblique fractures of

the mid one third femur, or of the mid one third of tibia in cases where internal fixation might be indicated, and also in the treatment of the vascular types of diaphyseal pseudarthrosis. The A.O. intramedullary nail, like the Kuentscher nail, is cloverleaf. However, the whole instrumentation, as well as the nail itself, is more refined and superior.

APPLICATIONS

The successful treatment of any fracture depends on many factors. Nicoll[4] coined the term "personality of the fracture" to outline these factors. Also of paramount importance is environment and the personnel involved in treatment. A careful study of these factors is of prime importance in choosing the best method of treatment.

If open means are the method of choice, one must first assess the operability of the fracture by all available means, both clinical and radiologic. Some fractures defy operative fixation even by the most skilled hands. Opening a fracture that cannot be stabilized destroys all soft tissue hinges, causes more trauma to the fracture site, and thereby gives one an inadequately fixed fracture that requires lengthy external immobilization. Better results can be achieved in these cases by using traction methods with early motion or cast bracing or both. Many of the operative techniques involved are difficult. The line diagrams in this chapter and in the A.O. manual do not convey the difficulty of the surgical techniques, and one should not be lured into a false sense of security by these diagrams.

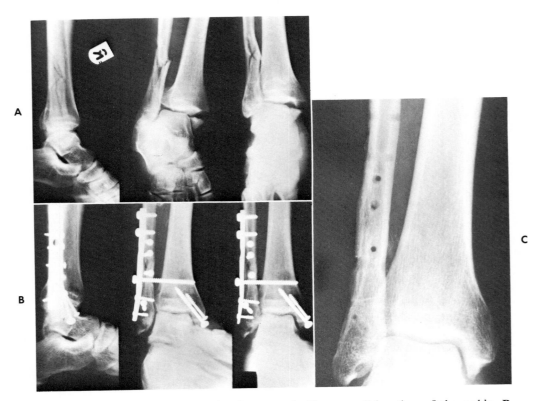

Fig. 3-14. Displaced intra-articular fracture. **A,** Fracture dislocation of the ankle. **B,** Following open reduction and internal fixation. **C,** At 1 year following removal of implant.

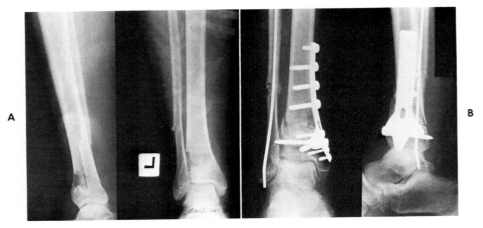

Fig. 3-15. A, Note large gap in metaphysis of this low "boot top" fracture, which appeared once reduction was carried out. **B,** After reduction, bone grafting of the defect, and internal fixation.

INDICATIONS

The following cases constitute our prime indications for open reduction.

Intra-articular fractures. These difficult fractures, especially of weight-bearing joints, must be carefully analyzed to be certain that it is technically possible to fix the fracture. If one fails to do so, one will have destroyed the chance of using traction successfully because of the division of soft tissue hinges. One will have devitalized bone, added to the trauma, and exposed the patient to the threat of sepsis. The physician should also be wary of the extremely comminuted fracture in the elderly, since their bone often is not strong enough to hold a screw. Displaced intra-articular fractures in young patients are the prime indication for open reduction (Fig. 3-14).

Metaphyseal fractures. When closed reduction of these fractures, especially those in the lower extremity with marked compression, bone loss, and displacement (Fig. 3-15), is attempted, a large gap often results. Healing is not only often delayed, but also the axial deformity often recurs. These fractures are best treated by open reduction, bone grafting, and application of a buttress plate. Again be very wary of these fractures in the elderly because of osteoporosis. If forced into an open reduction in a patient with severe osteoporosis, one may occasionally supplement the holding power of a crucial screw with bone cement to correct an almost impossible situation (Fig. 3-6).

Select diaphyseal fractures. In spite of the recent work on functional bracing of forearm fractures, we still believe that fractures of both bones of the forearm, isolated fractures of the ulna, and Monteggia or Galeazzi fracture dislocations are best treated by open reduction. All studies have shown that when this method is applied correctly, patients can discard all external splints at the end of 7 to 10 days, and most sedentary workers are back to full-time work within a month. Full return of function is the usual end result.

Fractures of the upper and middle third of the femur are a relative indication for open reduction. Although we recognize that fractures of the femur are managed by skeletal traction or cast bracing in many centers, we still feel that especially in upper and middle third fractures open reduction is the preferred method of treatment.

Tibial shaft fractures are rarely treated by open reduction. Surgery is reserved for difficult fractures entering a joint, where a satisfactory closed reduction cannot be obtained or maintained, or other rare circumstances.

Fractures of the humerus are rarely treated by open reduction. The indication here is often multiple fractures where internal fixation is carried out to facilitate nursing or where the fracture is associated with a vascular injury.

Complications of fractures. This method is invaluable in the treatment of complications of fractures including malunions, delayed union, and nonunion, both in infected and noninfected cases.

Other indications. Multiple diaphyseal fractures in one limb are a relative indication for open reduction in order to avoid problems such as the "floating knee syndrome" associated with ipsilateral femoral and tibial shaft fractures. The results of conservative treatment have proven less than satisfactory in these cases. The fixation of one or more fractures in a multiple injury patient facilitates nursing care. Although it was recently questioned in the Viet Nam experience, we still feel that fractures complicated by neurovascular injury are best treated by internal fixation.

Open fractures. We feel that a paradox exists in analyzing some of the dogmatic statements resulting from the Viet Nam experience with regard to implants in compound wounds. First, the most severe open injury one can receive is seen in traumatic amputation, yet the first principle in reimplanting the limb is stable internal fixation of the fracture. We feel that major open wounds including avulsion skin flaps and muscle loss are relative indications for internal fixation of fractures. We feel strongly, however, that soft tissue should then be handled in a like manner whether internal fixation is used or not, that is, careful cleansing of the wound, excision of devitalized tissue, and leaving the skin open where indicated. In our experience this has allowed rapid rehabilitation of the limb, reduced swelling, especially in avulsion skin flaps, and decreased the infection rate. We stress, however, that a high degree of surgical judgment is required in these cases. Stable fixation of open fractures is perhaps one of the most effective prophylactic measures against sepsis. However, if any doubt exists as to the degree of contamination or soft tissue viability, this fixation is best accomplished by the new types of rigid external fixators such as the Hoffmann or the A.O. tubular systems.

CONCLUSIONS

We feel that A.O. has made a valuable contribution to fracture care during the past 20 years. We do not feel that closed methods of fracture care should be abandoned. On the contrary, we use "functional casts" and braces with early weight bearing for tibia fractures, some femoral bracing techniques, and all the other armamentaria available to us. The astute surgeon will carefully examine each case and assign to that case "its own fracture personality." Based on the clinician's experience and personal expertise, the best treatment usually becomes obvious. If internal fixation seems the best treatment, then we recommend the A.O. system as a superb method of internal fixation. We feel, however, that the principles previously discussed should not be violated if external forms of splintage are to be abandoned and early motion started. The strength of this system is only as good as the bone in which it is placed. If at the end of the surgical procedure one is concerned about the strength of the bone, then some type of cast brace that allows early motion is preferable to jeopardizing the fixation and letting the fracture fall apart. Successful fracture treatment is a blend of the surgeon's skill and the best of both the closed and open methods of fracture care.

REFERENCES

1. Charnley, J.: Compression arthrodesis, Edinburgh, 1953, E. & S. Livingstone.
2. Danis, R.: In Müller, M. E., Allgöwer, M., and Willenegger, H., editors: Manual of internal fixation, New York, 1970, Springer Publishing Co., Inc., p. 10.
3. Key, J. A.: Positive pressure in arthrodesis for tuberculosis of the knee joint, South. Med. J. **25:**1932.
4. Nicoll, E. A.: Fractures of the tibial shaft, vol. 36B, 1964, pp. 373-387.
5. Perren, S. M., Huggler, A., Russenberger, M., Allgöwer, M., Mathys, R., Schenk, R. K., Willenegger, H., and Müller, M. E.: The reaction of cortical bone to compression, Acta Orthop. Scand. (Suppl), **125:**19, 1969.
6. Schatzker, J., Horne, J. G., and Summer-Smith, G.: The effects of movement on the holding power of screws in bone, Clin. Orthop. **111:**263, 1975.
7. Schenk, R. K., and Willenegger, H.: Zum histologischen Bild der sogennanten Primärheilung der Knochenkompakta nach experimentallen osteotomien am Hund, Experientia **19:**593, 1963.
8. Wagner, H.: Die Einbettung von Metallschrauben im Knochen und die Heilungsvorgänge des Knochengewebes unter dem Einfluss der stabilen Osteosynthese, Langenbecks Arch. Chir. **305:**28, 1963.

Chapter 4

Management of unstable pathologic fractures—dislocations of the spine and acetabulum, secondary to metastatic malignancy

KEVIN D. HARRINGTON

During the past 10 years, the recorded incidence of malignancy metastatic to the skeleton has increased steadily, and the frequency of pathologic fractures of the long bones, pelvis, and spine has increased as well. This phenomenon is a direct reflection of more aggressive and effective palliative treatment of patients with known metastases and those with a high risk for development of metastases. Treatment includes the use of combinations of hormonal manipulation, chemotherapy, and radiotherapy. In addition, the adjunctive use of methyl methacrylate to achieve more secure internal fixation of long bone fractures has allowed over 80% of these patients to regain an ambulatory status.[16]

Between 1960 and 1970, the published mean survival rate for patients following their first long bone pathologic fracture was 7.2 months.* At the present time, the figure has risen to 18.8 months.[16] When analyzed by primary origin, those patients suffering pathologic long bone fractures from metastatic carcinoma of the breast had a mean survival of 22.6 months, and those with primary carcinomas in the prostate gland and kidneys had mean survivals of 29.3 and 11.8 months, respectively. In contrast, patients with lung carcinomas still have a mean survival of only 3.6 months.

---

*See references 12, 16, 22, 23, 29, and 30.

The technique for surgical management of pathologic long bone fractures has been standardized.[15,16] The diseased bone and tumor tissue are resected and replaced by methyl methacrylate and supplemented by metal internal fixation devices or prostheses, the combination having a structural capacity to withstand the stresses of immediate weight bearing. The immediate efficacy of such fixation, as well as its long-term security, are well documented.[16]

Encouraged by such success with long bone fractures, clinicians have recently focused attention on attempts to apply the same fixation principles to the technically more demanding fractures that occur in the axial skeleton. Metastatic lesions of the spine and pelvis infrequently progress to fractures of sufficient severity to require internal fixation. However, when fixation is necessary, the orthopaedic surgeon is faced with the challenging paradox of bone subjected to high compression loads, yet of sufficiently small size and fragile composition to render the use of strong metal fixation devices technically impossible.

PATHOLOGIC FRACTURE-DISLOCATIONS OF THE SPINE

A patient with a metastatic malignancy involving the spine normally experiences slowly progressive local pain that can be relieved by irradia-

51

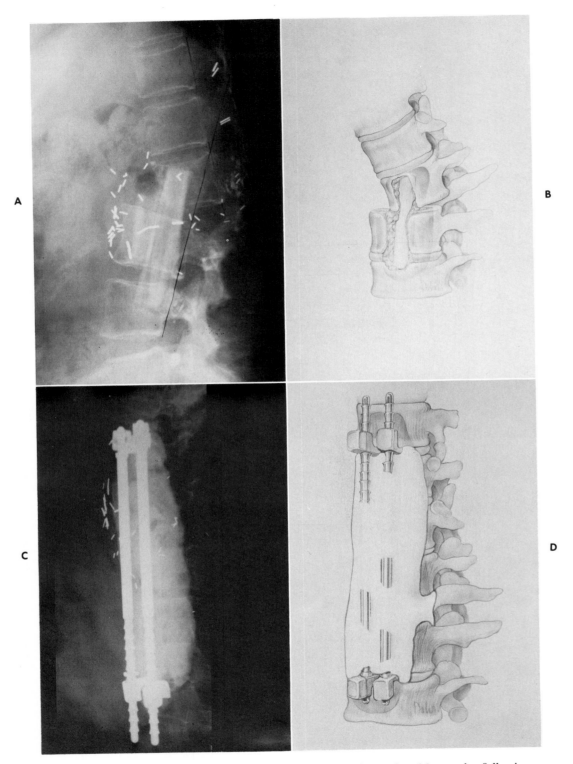

Fig. 4-1. A, Lateral roentgenogram of the thoracolumbar spine 36 months following T11-L3 laminectomy and 13 months after attempted anterior stabilization with iliac and rib bone grafts. The L2 vertebral body essentially is absent, and the body of L1 is dislocated posteriorly on L3. The spine is markedly unstable, and the bone grafts show no evidence of incorporation. **B,** Schematic representation of **A. C,** Anterior stabilization from T10-L4 was accomplished using methyl methacrylate and reinforced by Harrington distraction rods. **D,** Schematic representation of **C.**

tion. In some instances, rapidly destructive lesions may cause collapse of one or more vertebrae, with severe pain, increasing local kyphosis, and eventual neurologic deficits. None of these complications can be managed successfully by irradiation alone.[24,37] In fact, the early hyperemic response of the tissues to radiation may actually increase the risk of further compression of the vertebral body, resulting in worsening kyphosis.[24,26]

Conventional laminectomy decompression in such instances must be condemned because it rarely improves neurologic function. It often results in spinal instability with increasing kyphos because the remaining posterior stability of the spine has been surgically ablated in the face of disruption of anterior stability by the metastatic tumor process* (Fig. 4-1, *A* and *B*). Anterior decompression by resection of tumor and devitalized bone has proven effective because it relieves the cord or root impingement at its anterior source. Such impingement is a slowly progressive process not unlike that seen with tuberculosis and similarly destructive inflammatory processes involving the vertebrae.[18] The quadriplegia or paraplegia resulting from such a slowly progressive process is very responsive to anterior decompression, and, unlike the situation of acute traumatic cord lesions, a high incidence of neurologic improvement or recovery can be anticipated.

Moreover, the anterior approach enhances the efficacy of subsequent radiation therapy by markedly reducing the volume of tumor tissue and devitalized bone to; be irradiated.[5] Correction of spinal alignment and stabilization can be performed during the same operation.[18,19]

However, if stabilization is accomplished by bone grafting, immediate spinal stability is not achieved. Prolonged support by halo fixation or rigid neck bracing is required during healing, and the graft usually must be augmented by posterior stabilization and fusion.† In order to avoid interference and incorporation of bone grafts, postoperative irradiation ordinarily is either avoided or minimized, resulting in a high incidence of local tumor recurrence.[10,31,37,39]

Attempts have been made to achieve instantaneous spinal stability by augmenting conventional wiring of the posterior elements with methyl methacrylate applied over the laminae.[3,32,36] This technique shares with laminectomy the disadvantage of attempting to decompress a lesion in front of the neural elements via an approach from behind those elements. The method has been successful in mechanically stabilizing the spine in the absence of any major vertebral bone loss.[3,32,36] However, even with inherent stability afforded by an intact vertebral body, the fixation achieved is subject to failure at the ends of the acrylic and wire mass with forces as low (70 newtons) as those caused by simple forward flexion.[28] When anterior instability exists because of destruction of the vertebral bodies, much lower forces are required to cause failure by sheer or kyphotic angulation.[20]

Scoville[32] first demonstrated the feasibility of anterior vertebral resection and replacement-stabilization using methyl methacrylate in dog experiments and, later, in a single patient with a lymphoma destroying two cervical vertebrae. The technique incorporates the advantages of a direct anterior approach to the tumor mass for effective decompression of the neural or vascular elements together with the potential for achieving immediate mechanical spinal stability not dependent on bony healing or adversely affected by radiation.

Almost invariably, such patients experience severe pain at the vertebral fracture site. The majority also manifest a significant neurologic involvement preoperatively. Most often, fractures of the cervical spine require operative intervention, not only because of the frequency of metastatic involvement there, but also because the relatively small intraspinal space tolerates minimal impingement on the cord or roots before significant neurologic deficit develops.

Because vertebral involvement by metastases usually is recognized before neurologic impingement becomes apparent, patients ordinarily have been irradiated before surgical decompression, and stabilization is considered. The mean dose employed in our experience is 4775 rad.

Operative technique

The operative technique involves resection of all tumorous and structurally inadequate bone (Fig. 4-2, and *A* and *B*) and, in instances of neurologic involvement, exposure of adjacent neural elements for decompression. In most instances, the anterior longitudinal ligament is found to be intact but grossly discolored and bulging at the

---

*See references 1, 4-6, 21, 37, 41, and 42.
†See references 10, 19, 31, 33, 37, and 38.

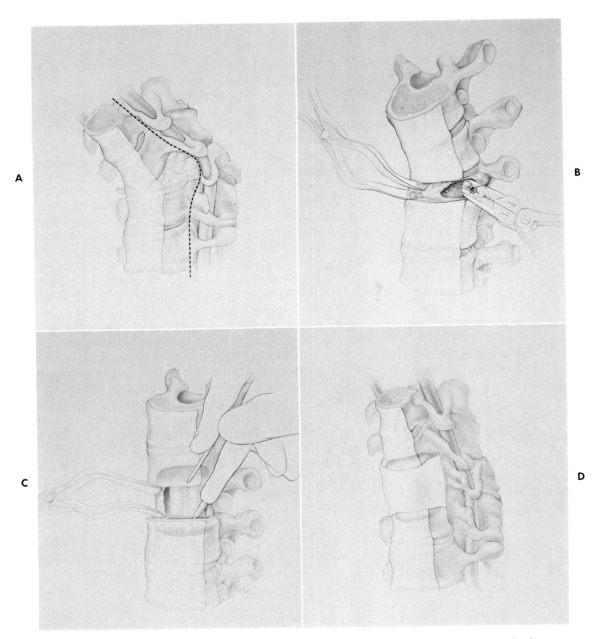

Fig. 4-2. A, Replacement of vertebral body by tumor results in the collapse of the body, increasing kyphus and the extrusion of the tumor and bony fragments into the epidural space. **B,** With the use of a lamina spreader, the vertebral space is reconstructed anteriorly. The tumor is resected using a rongeur and curettes. **C,** Once the vertebral space has been restored and neural elements completely exposed and decompressed, endplates of adjacent vertebrae are opened with a power bur, and the bone is undercut to enhance fixation of the methyl methacrylate. **D,** The prosthetic vertebral body reconstituting the normal vertebral height and correcting the kyphotic deformity.

tumor site with the fracture level thus easily identifiable.

The anterior longitudinal ligament is removed locally by sharp dissection, and the level of the collapsed vertebra clearly defined by curettage. A lamina spreader is used to restore the normal vertebral space, thereby correcting any associated kyphotic deformities (Fig. 4-2, *B*). Any residual disc material is resected, and the end plates of the adjacent vertebrae undercut with a power burr to promote fixation of the acrylic and minimize the risk of displacement of the methyl methacrylate mass after polymerization (Fig. 4-2, *C*).

With the exception of the single multilevel replacement augmented by anterior Harrington rods (Fig. 4-1, *C* and *D*), no ancillary fixation or replacement materials have been necessary. The acrylic simply acts as a filler to maintain the vertebral space under tension, and the solidarity of the fixation depends on the tensional rigidity of the remaining soft tissues and spinal posterior elements (Fig. 4-2, *D*).

It has been demonstrated experimentally[40] that there are no adverse thermal or chemical effects of the polymerizing cement on the neural elements. This is probably because the cerebrospinal fluid circulating within the intact dural space acts as an effective heat sink, thereby protecting the spinal cord and nerve roots. Nevertheless, great care must be taken to prevent impingement by the expanding acrylic mass on cord or root structures and to separate the cement mass from the underlying dura by a layer of Gelfoam.

Barium-impregnated methyl methacrylate is used in order to enhance radiologic identification of the position of the cement postoperatively. There is no evidence that the presence of methyl methacrylate interferes with local irradiation therapy,[14,16] nor does irradiation weaken or otherwise alter the cement.[8,27] Postoperatively, patients need use only brief soft support (cervical collar or corset).

In my experience, there have been no instances of local tumor recurrence either in soft tissue or bony elements. No neurologic complications have occurred, and no patients have deteriorated neurologically postoperatively. Failure of stabilization has occurred in one instance because extensive destruction of vertebral bone throughout the cervical spine made it impossible to achieve secure fixation of the acrylic replacement mass. Obviously, such a situation should be anticipated, if possible, before a patient is subjected to such surgical intervention.

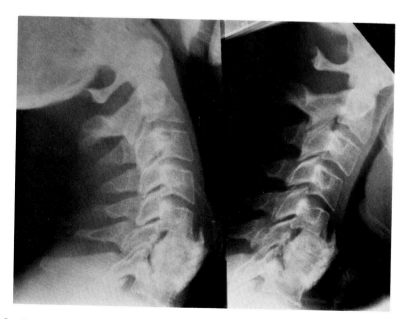

Fig. 4-3. Postoperative flexion-extension roentgenograms obtained 9 months after replacement-stabilization at C6. Little if any motion is demonstrable at the "fusion" site. The patient's neck was asymptomatic.

The great majority of patients have benefited from the procedure with sustained relief of local fracture pain. In our experience, almost all the patients with neurologic involvement have demonstrated marked improvement postoperatively. Patients who had undergone conventional laminectomy before the stabilization procedure showed neurologic deterioration as often as improvement, and most also suffered from an increase in the local kyphotic deformity. After anterior stabilization with acrylic, however, the patients realized improvement in or recovery of neurologic function together with relief from local mechanical spine pain and sustained restitution of spinal stability.

Flexion-extension roentgenograms obtained postoperatively have revealed no significant motion across the acrylic-bone interface, reflecting the solidity of the "fusion" apparent clinically (Fig. 4-3).

ACETABULAR FRACTURES

The displaced pathologic acetabular fracture secondary to metastases presents a combination of therapeutic problems for the orthopaedic surgeon that are the culmination of two destruction processes leading to joint instability. These processes are (1) the phenomenon of tumor and radiation osteolysis, which results in gradual acetabular protrusion, and (2) the specific fracture disrupting the integrity of the joint surface. The loss of periacetabular bone resulting from both processes seriously interferes with attempts at joint stabilization or reconstruction.

Problems specific to osteolysis

When analyzed separately, the protrusio acetabuli (Fig. 4-4) is comparable to the same deformity caused by benign inflammatory or osteolytic processes unrelated to metastatic disease.[11,25,35] The femoral head tends to migrate

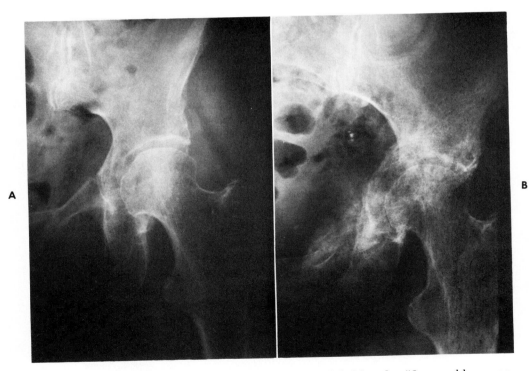

Fig. 4-4. A, Anteroposterior roentgenogram of the left hip of a 52-year-old woman with metastatic carcinoma of the rectum. Lytic infiltration of the medial acetabular wall with a minimally displaced fracture is apparent. **B,** Six weeks later, after the completion of local irradiation (4000 rad) more extensive lysis and softening of the bone is apparent with displacement of the femoral head. Protrusio has resulted from softening of the bone caused by a combination of tumor lysis and postirradiation hyperemia.

both medially and superiorly in accordance with the normal stress forces across the hip joint.[11]

Conventional efforts to arrest the process have included bone grafting of the medial acetabular wall, valgus osteotomy of the femur, and total hip replacement using specialized prostheses and augmented by a reinforcing bone graft or methyl methacrylate.[25,35]

However, acetabular protrusion secondary to metastatic disease differs from the more benign type of protrusio because of the necessity to irradiate the tumor site to control progressive bone destruction. Radiation, in conventional dosage of 4000 to 6000 rad, seriously reduces the likelihood that bone grafted for reinforcement of the acetabular wall will ever be incorporated. The healing of an osteotomy of the adjacent proximal femur thus also is endangered. The protrusio

process often accelerates dramatically as a direct result of the hyperemia and osteitis caused by irradiation itself.[13]

Problems specific to the fracture

Loss of articular congruity as a result of direct tumor lysis (Fig. 4-5) or of disruption by a fracture-dislocation prevents the possibility of obtaining a pain-free hip except by resection of the femoral head, amputation of the limb or a portion of the pelvis, or prosthetic replacement.

Ablation of the joint by resectioning of the proximal femur or hemipelvis has been advocated by many, particularly where extensive tumor osteolysis exists.[9,15] Enneking[9] recommended that hip fusion be attempted even after wide resectioning of the acetabular bone for primary malignancy but emphasized that a successful, pain-free

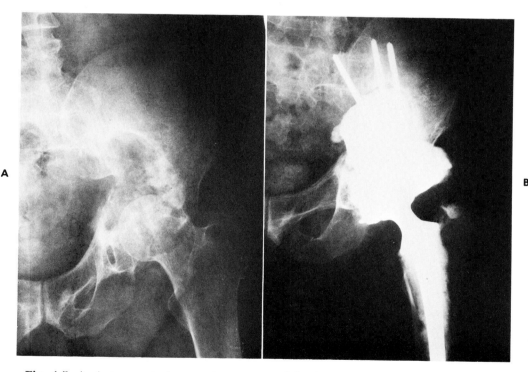

Fig. 4-5. A, Anteroposterior roentgenogram of the left hip of a 51-year-old man with metastatic carcinoma of the adrenal cortex. Extensive lytic destruction of the supra-acetabular bone is apparent with migration of the femoral head proximally. **B,** Eighteen months after resection of the destroyed bone and tumor and hip replacement. The acetabular component remains securely fixed to the pelvis by a combination of threaded Steinman pins, wire mesh, protrusio shell, and methyl methacrylate cement. The lucent halo above the cement mass was apparent from the time of surgery. Absence of apparent loosening of the fixation pins attests to the stability of fixation.

fusion occurred in less than half the cases where it was attempted. In any event, prosthetic reconstruction of a stable hip generally is considered a preferable alternative to ablation or fusion.

In those cases where no significant displacement of the femoral head has occurred, total hip replacement arthroplasty can be performed with anticipation of achieving a stable and pain-free joint. Sim[34] reported on 35 cases of hip joint replacement after a pathologic fracture of the proximal femur in patients with minimal, if any, involvement of the periacetabular bone. He encountered no difficulties in effectively securing the acetabular component, and his results were excellent with regard to joint stability and relief of pain.

However, where major displacement of the femoral head has occurred, conventional total hip replacement is likely to fail because there is insufficient structurally adequate bone around the acetabular component to prevent its loosening and migration.

The problem of inadequate bone stock

Insufficiency of bone stock of the medial acetabular wall will encourage medial migration of the total hip components unless the acetabular portion can be buttressed against bone with adequate structural integrity (Fig. 4-6). As already noted, attempting to reinforce the medial wall by bone grafting is impractical in the face of anticipated radiation of the joint.

Harris and Oh[25] have designed a chrome-cobalt protrusio shell that effectively diverts stress against the acetabular component of a total hip away from the weakened or deficient medial acetabular wall and onto the lateral acetabular rim by means of phalanges built into the shell (Fig. 4-7, *D*).

Insufficiency of bone stock of the acetabular roof presents a much more difficult challenge. Attempts to deepen the acetabulum medially in order to gain a wider roof result in weakening and often late fatigue fractures of the medial wall. Attempts to deepen the acetabular roof superiorly in order to gain an effective buttress result in failure because the ilial wing above the normal acetabular roof is thin and inadequate to securely support the combination of acrylic cement and prosthetic acetabular component (Fig. 4-7, *A* and *B*).

Reconstructing the superior acetabular bone stock by splitting the ilium, acetabuloplasties of the Chiari or shelf type, or using the femoral head to bone graft the deficient area have been successful in the management of congenital acetabular insufficiency unrelated to malignancy.[2,7,17] However, in the face of postoperative irradiation, all such techniques that depend on healing of osteotomized or grafted bone must be anticipated to fail.

The solution to insufficiency of bone stock in the acetabular rim or roof lies in transmitting the weight-bearing forces superomedially away from the periacetabular bone destroyed by tumor and into the bone of the ilium and sacrum still structurally intact (Fig. 4-7, *C* to *E*).

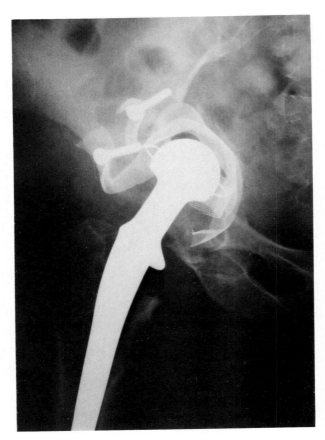

Fig. 4-6. Anteroposterior roentgenogram of the right hip in a patient undergoing hip replacement for a pathologic fracture of the medial acetabular wall. The surgeon attempted to achieve fixation of the acetabular component by a combination of mesh and methyl methacrylate alone. Medial and superior migration of the component has occurred.

Operative techniques

Displaced pathologic fractures of the acetabulum must be subdivided into two classes, depending on the adequacy of bone stock in the acetabular rim and roof.

Class I fractures include those with destruction of bone confined to the *medial* acetabular wall, but with the acetabular rim and major portion of the roof intact (Fig. 4-6). These are managed by conventional total hip replacement reinforced by

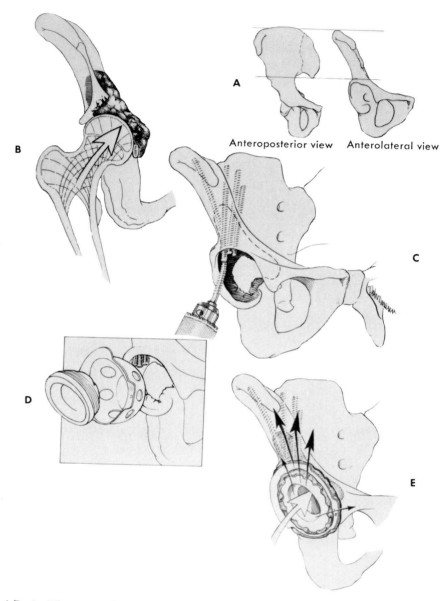

Anteroposterior view   Anterolateral view

Fig. 4-7. A, The anterolateral view of pelvis demonstrates the thinness of the ilium superior to the acetabulum. **B,** Tumor has destroyed the superior and medial acetabular bone, leaving minimal intact cortex for fixation of the acetabular component. **C,** After tumor tissue is resected, Steinman pins can be drilled from the periacetabular cavity into the structurally sound bone of the superior ilium and across the sacroiliac joint. **D,** The acetabular component as it sits in the protrusio shell. **E.** The combination of acetabular cup, protrusio shell, and Steinman pins incorporated into methyl methacrylate effectively transmits weight-bearing stresses into strong bone of the ilial wing and sacrum.

the Harris-Oh protrusio shell, which transmits the majority of weight-bearing stress against the intact acetabular rim. Chrome-cobalt mesh is used in addition to reinforce the deficient medial wall and to minimize the escape of methyl methacrylate within the pelvis (Fig. 4-5, *B*).

Class II fractures include those with loss of structural integrity of the bone of the acetabular *roof and/or rim* (Figs. 4-4, *A*, and 4-5, *A*). In these cases, the tumor tissue and destroyed bone are curetted widely until sufficiently strong bone deep within the iliac wing is reached. Large, threaded Steinman pins then are drilled proximally from the acetabulum into the intact bone of the ilium and across the sacroiliac joint into the lateral sacral wing (Fig. 4-7, *C*). The protrusio shell is again used, and a combination of acetabular component, shell, mesh, and Steinman pins is fixed securely used methyl methacrylate (Fig. 4-7, *D* and *E*). The result is a rigid combination of materials similar in concept to reinforced concrete wherein the stresses of weightbearing are transmitted into structurally intact bone of the upper pelvis and sacrum.

Aims of surgery

When considering whether to attempt stabilization and reconstruction of the hip joint in such instances, the orthopaedic surgeon must evaluate a hierarchy of surgical aims to be weighed against the risks of the procedure itself. In descending order of importance, one must consider carefully whether the following possibilities can be realized:
1. Achieving lasting relief of hip pain
2. Regaining stability of the hips sufficient for weight-bearing ambulation
3. Regaining sufficient hip motion to allow easy resumption of normal activities of daily living
4. Positioning and stabilizing the hip to allow effective function of normal surrounding musculature
5. Restoring limb length
6. Creating a biomechanically sound joint system unlikely to fail in the face of prolonged or repeated stress anticipated for long-term survivors.

In appropriately selected patients, the techniques outlined here have successfully fulfilled these criteria, and the reconstructed hips have continued to function during follow-up periods of as long as five years without failure.

REFERENCES

1. Arseni, C. N., Simionescu, M. D., and Horwath, L.: Tumors of the spine, a follow-up study of 350 patients with neurosurgical considerations, Acta Psychiatr. Neurol. Scand. **34:** 398, 1959.
2. Aufranc, O. E.: Constructive surgery of the hip, St. Louis, 1962, The C. V. Mosby Co.
3. Bernhang, A. M., Rosen, H., and Leivy, D.: Internal methyl methacrylate splint, Orthop. Rev. **7:**25, 1978.
4. Brice, J., and McKissoch, W.: Surgical treatment of malignant extradural spinal tumors, Br. Med. J. **1:**1341, 1965.
5. Bucy, P. C.: The treatment of malignant tumors of the spine: a review, Neurology **13:**938, 1963.
6. Callahan, R. A., Johnson, R. M., Margolis, R. N., Keggi, K. J., Albright, J. A., and Southwick, W. O.: Cervical facet fusion for control of instability following laminectomy, J. Bone Joint Surg. **59-A:**991, 1977.
7. Colton, C. L.: Chiari osteotomy for acetabular dysplasia in young subjects, J. Bone Joint Surg. **54-B:**548, 1972.
8. Eftekhar, N. D., and Thurston, C. W.: Effect of irradiation on acrylic cement with special reference to fixation of pathological fractures, J. Biomech. **8:**53, 1975.
9. Enneking, W. F., and Durham, W. K.: Resection and reconstruction for primary neoplasms involving the innominate bone, J. Bone Joint Surg. **60-A:**731, 1978.
10. Fielding, J. W., Pyle, R. N., and Fietti, V. G.: Anterior cervical vertebral body resection and bone grafting for benign and malignant tumors, J. Bone Joint Surg. **61-A:**251, 1979.
11. Frankel, V. H., and Burstein, A. H.: Orthopedic biomechanics, Philadelphia, 1976, Lea & Febiger, p. 27.
12. Galasko, C. S. B.: Pathological fractures secondary to metastatic cancer, J. R. Coll. Surg. **19:**351, 1974.
13. Hall, F. M., Mauch, P. M., Levine, M. B., and Goldstein, M. A.: Protrusio acetabuli following pelvic irradiation, Am. J. Radiology **132:**291, 1979.
14. Harrington, K. D.: The use of methyl methacrylate as an adjunct in the internal fixation of unstable comminuted intertrochanteric fractures in osteoporotic patients, J. Bone Joint Surg. **57-A:**744, 1975.
15. Harrington, K. D., Johnston, J. O., Turner, R. H., and Green, D. L.: The use of methyl methacrylate as an adjunct in the internal fixation of malignant neoplastic fractures, J. Bone Joint Surg. **54-A:**1665, 1972.
16. Harrington, K. D., Sim, F. H., Enis, J. E., Johnston, J. O., Dick, H. M., and Gristina, A. G.: Methyl methacrylate as an adjunct in the internal fixation of pathological fractures, J. Bone Joint Surg. **58-A:**1047, 1976.
17. Harris, W. H., and Crothers, O. D.: Autogenous bone grafting using the femoral head to correct severe acetabular deficiency for total hip replacement. In The hip, vol. 4, St. Louis, 1976, The C. V. Mosby Co.
18. Hodgson, A. R., and Stock, F. E.: Anterior spine fusion for the treatment of tuberculosis of the spine, J. Bone Joint Surg. **42-A:**295, 1960.
19. Jenkins, D. H. R.: Extensive cervical laminectomy—long-term results, Br. J. Surg., **60:**852, 1973.
20. Johnston, J. O.: Unpublished data, 1979.
21. Kennady, J. C., and Stern, W. E.: Metastatic neoplasms of the vertebral column producing compression of the spinal cord, Am. J. Surg. **104:**155, 1962.

22. Koskinen, E. V., and Nieminen, R. A.: Surgical treatment of metastatic pathological fractures of major long bones, Acta Orthop. Scand. **44:**539, 1973.

23. Marcove, R. C., and Yang, D. J.: Survival times after treatment of pathologic fractures, Cancer **20:**2154, 1967.

24. Martin, N. S., and Williamson, J.: The role of surgery in the treatment of malignant tumors of the spine, J. Bone Joint Surg. **52-B:**227, 1970.

25. McCollum, D. E., and Nunley, J. A.: Bone grafting in acetabular protrusio: a biologic buttress. In The hip, vol. 6, St. Louis, 1978, The C. V. Mosby Co.

26. Mullan, J., and Evans, J. P.: Neoplastic disease of the spinal extradural space, Arch. Surg. **74:**900, 1957.

27. Murray, J. A., Bruels, M. C., and Lindberg, R. D.: Irradiation of polymethylmethacrylate. In vitro gamma radiation effect, J. Bone Joint Surg. **56-A:**311, 1974.

28. Panjabi, M. M., Hopper, W., White, A. A., and Keggi, K. J.: Posterior spine stabilization with methyl methacrylate, Spine **2:**241, 1977.

29. Parrish, F. F., and Murray, J. A.: Surgical treatment for secondary neoplastic fractures. A retrospective study of ninety-six patients, J. Bone Joint. Surg. **52-A:**665, 1970.

30. Perez, C. A., Bradfield, J. S., and Morgan, H. C.: Management of pathologic fractures, Cancer **79:**648, 1972.

31. Raycroft, J. F., Hochman, R. P., and Southwick, W. D.: Metastatic tumors involving the cervical vertebrae: surgical palliation, J. Bone Joint Surg. **60-A:**763, 1978.

32. Scoville, W. B., Palmer, A. H., Samra, K., and Chong, G.: The use of acrylic plastic for vertebral replacement or fixation in metastatic disease of the spine, J. Neurosurg. **27:**274, 1967.

33. Seres, J. L.: Fusion in the presence of severe metastatic destruction of the cervical spine (case report), J. Neurosurg. **28:**592, 1968.

34. Sim, F. H., Hartz, C. R., and Chao, E. Y. S.: Total hip arthroplasty for tumors of the hip. In The hip, vol. 4, St. Louis, 1976, The C. V. Mosby Co.

35. Sotelo-Garza, A., and Charnley, J.: The results of Charnley arthroplasty of the hip performed for protrusio acetabuli, Clin. Orthop. **132:**12, 1978.

36. Spence, W. T.: Internal plastic splint for stabilization of the spine, Clin. Orthop. **92:**325, 1973.

37. Stener, B.: Complete removal of three vertebrae for giant cell tumor, J. Bone Joint Surg. **53-B:**278, 1971.

38. Stener, B.: Total spondylectomy in chondrosarcoma arising from the seventh thoracic vertebra, J. Bone Joint Surg. **53-B:**288, 1971.

39. Streitz, W., Brown, J. C., and Bonnett, C. A.: Anterior fibular strut grafting in the treatment of kyphosis, Clin. Orthop. **128:**140, 1977.

40. Wang, G. J., Reger, S. I., McLaughlin, R. E., Stamp, W. G., and Albin, D.: Safety of cement fixation in cervical spine (studies of a rabbit model), unpublished data, 1978.

41. White, A. H., and Wiltse, L. L.: Spondylolisthesis after extensive lumbar laminectomy, J. Bone Joint Surg. **58-A:**727, 1976.

42. Wright, R. L.: Malignant tumors in the spinal extradural space: results of surgical treatment, Ann. Surg. **157:**227, 1963.

Chapter 5

Injuries to the growth plate and the epiphysis

ROBERT S. SIFFERT

Although there exist many biochemical and enzymatic unknowns regarding chondrogenesis and osteogenesis, there is abundant physiologic, anatomic experimental,[16] and morphologic information to serve as the basis for understanding the effects of trauma on growth cartilage. Salter and Harris[49] analyzed clinical and experimental injuries to the growth plate and classified their mechanisms and patterns of healing and deformity as valuable guidelines for clinical management. This chapter will review briefly the mechanism of enchondral ossification at the longitudinal growth plate (LGP) and vertebrae and epiphysoid bones of the hand and foot as background for a discussion of the effects of injury to the epiphysis and growth plate. Details of current biochemical and enzymatic knowledge of growth cartilage activity, which are beyond the scope of this presentation, are well discussed in numerous reports and symposia in the current literature.*

The fetal model of adult bone is composed completely of growth cartilage except in the skull and clavicle, which grow by membranous ossification. The cartilage model expands principally by multiplication of chondroblasts on the surface (appositional growth) and production of a space-occupying cartilage matrix (interstitial growth). At a genetically predetermined time the cells in the center of the long bone cartilage model expand and degenerate, blood vessels invade, and the matrix calcifies, serving as the template for ossification, which is similar to the mechanism of enchondral ossification at a fracture site or at the metaphysis. The cartilaginous diaphysis is rapidly replaced by bone, and its perichondrium is transformed into a membranous bone forming periosteum. The bone-cartilage junction at either end of a long bone identifies the boundary between the metaphysis and the epiphysis. As the epiphysis enlarges appositionally and interstitially, the bony model grows circumferentially by periosteal bone formation and longitudinally by placement of cartilage at the newly organizing growth plate. Mankin[35] demonstrated that there appear to be two layers of germinal cells at the periphery of the epiphysis: an outer layer, which produces a thin gliding layer of surface cells and an inner layer, which gives rise to growth cartilage of the epiphysis itself.

A bony centrum appears within the epiphysis or epiphysoid bone in a manner similar to ossification of the long bone model (Fig. 5-1). As the bony nucleus enlarges, its vascularity is derived from the rich network of vessels preformed within the fetal epiphyseal cartilage matrix. The bony centrum replaces epiphyseal cartilage rapidly until a balance is established between the rate of appositional cartilage growth and ossification, maintaining a predictable and gradually decreasing volume of growth cartilage through adolescence. Distally, ossification ceases just short of the metaphysis, forming a dense bony end plate and leaving a thin layer of growth cartilage, which functions as the longitudinal growth plate (LGP) or physis until adult life. On the roentgenogram the LGP appears as a lucent area between two transverse dense lines, the bony end plate of the

---

*See references 7, 13, 14, 23, 24, 30, 37, 44, 54, 58, 64, and 66.

62

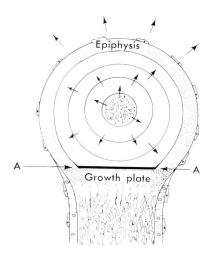

Fig. 5-1. Bony centrum of an epiphysis appears at a genetically predetermined site and time and enlarges to replace cartilage that is forming by appositional surface chondroblasts. When the bony centrum reaches the longitudinal growth plate, it condenses to form a horizontal bony end-plate *(A)*. The surrounding epiphyseal cartilage functions as a dome-shaped growth plate until adult life. At the superior and inferior surfaces of vertebrae, the growth plate is horizontal, and in epiphysoid bones of the hand and foot, it is spherical, completely surrounding the bony centrum. (From American Academy of Orthopaedic Surgeons: Instructional course lectures, vol. 22, St. Louis, 1973, The C. V. Mosby Co.)

epiphysis and the metaphyseal zone of ossification (new bone forming on calcified cartilage remnants as the primary spongiosa).

Nutrition to the LGP is derived from epiphyseal vessels that penetrate the bony end plate and the thin layers of subjacent reserve or resting cells to terminate as capillaries among the proliferating cartilage cells (Fig. 5-2). When adulthood is reached, the hormonal stimulus to growth fades, and cartilage cell proliferation ceases. As each layer of the plate matures and is not replenished, the plate itself narrows and is eventually replaced by metaphyseal bone until it is obliterated and union occurs between the metaphysis and the epiphysis. Slowing of growth is evident on the roentgenogram by narrowing of the plate. Cessation of growth is reflected by the presence of a single transverse dense line as the plate disappears and primary spongiosa contacts the bony end plate, rather than the double line of an actively growing LGP. Cancellous continuity is established between the epiphysis and metaphysis,

but a single transverse roentgen marker, which is a reflection of the circumferential cortical remnant of the bony end plate, may remain throughout life.

Nutrition to growing epiphyseal cells is derived from the following sources:

1. Joint fluid, which penetrates deeply into the cartilage mass,[15] facilitated by alternating pressure effects of normal joint motion
2. Large numbers of blood vessels distributed throughout the cartilage model[63]

THE GROWTH MECHANISM[13,44,54]

Except for appositional growth of the epiphysis, increase in long bone length occurs only in the zone of growth of the LGP (Fig. 5-2). Metabolic activities of cells within the zone of transformation then modify the matrix formed in the zone of growth to become calcifiable, elaborate calcium salts and produce dense longitudinally oriented collagen fibers, which offer mechanical support to the hypertrophying cells. Only when calcification within the matrix has occurred, do metaphyseal vascular loops invade and initiate the process of bone formation. In a patient with rickets, for example, the plate widens as a result of accumulation of newly forming cartilage, since orderly invasion of metaphyseal vessels is inhibited, and it returns to normal only after matrix calcification is restored. The zone of cartilage transformation consists of an incompletely understood sequence of metabolic processes (Fig. 5-2, *A*), including energy cycles, phosphorylization, calcification mechanisms, collagen synthesis, and eventually lysosomal and cellular complexes concerned with removal of remnants of the aging and necrotic cartilage cells.

The zone of ossification of the plate is much like a honeycomb lattice. Metaphyseal blood vessels channel into the spaces left by degenerating cartilage cells. Primary spongiosa of the metaphysis is then formed by osteoblasts, which are derived by metaplasia from endothelial buds and produce osteoid on the calcified cartilage lattice.

The process of cartilage growth, transformation, and then replacement by bone is similar at all sites of enchondral ossification. The gross morphologic configuration of this mechanism depends upon its anatomic location, being flat at the LGP and vertebral surfaces, dome-shaped in the epiphysis, and spheric in epiphysoid bones. Microscopically, it is a reflection of the speed of

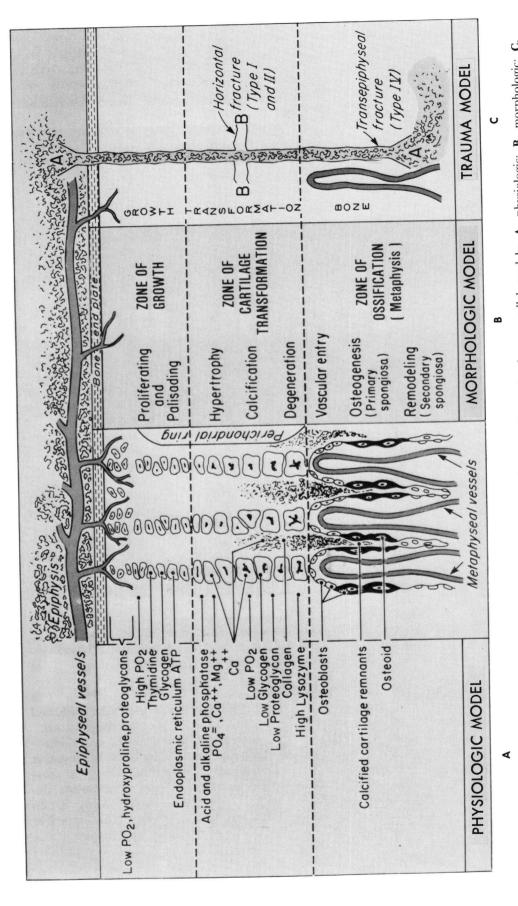

Fig. 5-2. Epiphyseal dynamics. Problems relating to the growth plate are shown in three parallel models: **A,** physiologic; **B,** morphologic; **C,** morphologic. All traumatic. Although growth represents a completely integrated process, the three morphologic zones have some degree of functional independence. All growth occurs only in the zone of growth. Factors that inhibit proliferation of cells (malnutrition, pressure) retard growth, and hyperemia results in growth stimulation. Irreparable damage produces growth arrest. The zone of cartilage transformation is concerned with (1) modifying the matrix, which collagen-was produced in the zone of growth so that it could be calcified, (2) the process of calcification, and (3) development of an intercellular, collagen supported, structural lattice. Injuries to this zone, most notably a horizontal fracture (Types I and II, *B* in the trauma model), do not interfere with the zone of growth, and growth continues. Vascularity to the zone of growth and cartilage transformation is derived from vessels in the epiphysis that penetrate the bony end-plate and the subjacent thin layer of reserve or resting cartilage cells to end in the area of proliferating and palisading cells. The zone of osteogenesis is concerned with formation of primary spongiosa. Osteoblasts derived from invading capillary buds produce osteoid and fibrillar bone on the honeycomb calcified cartilage lattice remnants of the plate. In the trauma model a longitudinal fracture that extends from the epiphysis to the metaphysis creates a potential channel for tethering bone formation and epiphysiodesis (A).

growth, being thinner and with fewer cells in each zone in the epiphysis, epiphysoid bones, and the vertebrae where growth is relatively slower than at the more rapidly enlarging longitudinal growth plate.

Functional models, constructed from the vast and increasing information available about growth cartilage, can serve as practical guides for the investigator, physician, and orthopaedic surgeon. For example, a physiologic model (Fig. 5-2, *A*) serves the requirements of the investigator, and a morphologic model (Fig. 5-2, *B*) serves the student and the clinician. Further simplification into a trauma model (Fig. 5-2, *C*) can assist the orthopaedist in understanding principles of practical management of the injured young patient. When the models are constructed in a horizontal fashion, ready access is available by cross-reference to all data that may be required for clinical decision-making. The trauma model will be used as the basis for this discussion of injuries to the growth plate and the epiphysis with appropriate references to the parallel physiologic and morphologic models.

Although the mechanism of enchondral ossification represents a smooth sequence of events, each depending upon the physiologic integrity of the preceding zone, there is a certain degree of independence about each zone that is important in understanding the pathophysiology and clinical principles of management of epiphyseal trauma.

Zone of growth

As long as normal vascularity to proliferating cells is unimpaired, cartilage cell multiplication generally continues unaffected at the longitudinal growth plate, regardless of traumatic or metabolic changes that might occur in the subsequent zones of transformation or ossification. Malnutrition and poor health, however, may result in inhibition of proliferating cells, probably mediated through lack of essential collagen and proteoglycan building blocks and alterations in growth hormone complexes. Within the epiphysis the vessels concerned with osteogenesis of the centrum also nourish the deeper layers of cartilage cells,[36] while at the zone of ossification of the LGP their sole function is to form bone. If vascularity to the bony nucleus is interrupted, appositional and interstitial epiphyseal cartilage growth of the outer layers continues, provided joint nutrition is maintained. Salter[47] demonstrated that deformity

did not occur following experimentally induced avascular necrosis of the femoral head in the pig. Epiphyseal cartilage cells continued to proliferate normally as the necrotic center became revascularized. These experimental findings correspond to those clinical circumstances where biomechanical forces remain undisturbed as in Köhler's disease of the tarsal navicular. At the hip, however, coxa magna[51] and subluxation,[55] which may accompany avascular necrosis of the femoral centrum in Legg-Calvé-Perthes syndrome, frequently lead to distortion of normal joint biomechanics and deformity. Current clinical management programs attempt to restore head-acetabular centration by bracing or surgery while at the same time maintaining growth cartilage nutrition by permitting normal joint motion and weight bearing (Fig. 5-7).

Irreparable injury or destruction of proliferating chondroblasts that may occur as a result of excessive sustained pressure within the growth plate or epiphysis[48,62] will result in permanent growth arrest and deformity. Moderate, sustained pressure, however, inhibits proliferation of cartilage cells.[5] Metabolic capabilities remain unimpaired,[20] and when pressure is relieved, growth resumes, which is often associated with a brief growth spurt. Early osteotomy to relieve abnormal medial pressure in tibia vara permits reconstitution of the depressed posteromedial articular surface of the epiphysis and resumption of medial growth at the LGP, and posterior soft tissue release of a foot and ankle contracture may correct a flat top talus.

In essence, therefore, the zone of growth is the heart of the growth plate mechanism. It is responsible for physical enlargement by production of cartilage cells and cartilage matrix. Since activities in the zone of growth are essentially independent of disorders or injuries that affect other areas of the plate, as long as the integrity of this zone is maintained, there is high probability of healing without deformity.

Zone of cartilage transformation

Transverse fractures of the growth plate generally occur through the zone of hypertrophic cells where immature calcified collagen-supported matrix is weakest.[49] This temporary disruption in the physiologic sequences within the zone of transformation also interrupts the continuous supply of calcified cartilage to metaphyseal vessels

(Fig. 5-2, *C*), thereby temporarily inhibiting ossification. There is no effect on growth cartilage proliferation, and the plate widens. Repair of a transverse fracture in the usual sense of fracture healing does not occur, but cartilage cells distal to the fracture apparently hypertrophy and degenerate and are replaced by metaphyseal osteogenesis until normal growth plate physiology is restored.

Alterations that may occur in physiologic functions within the zone of transformation that interfere with the process of manufacturing a calcifiable matrix, or calcification itself, do not impair osteogenic capabilities of the subsequent zone of ossification nor influence cell proliferation in the zone of growth. The few calcified remnants that become calcified in altered physiologic states (rickets) serve as a template for a new bone formation in the zone of ossification, producing a patchy and irregular primary spongiosa.

Zone of ossification

Injury to the osteogenic zone itself or the metaphysis does not affect longitudinal growth, cartilage transformation, or cartilage calcification. The plate widens as a result of accumulation of normally calcified cartilage and rapidly returns to normal when metaphyseal vascularity is restored.

The independent functional characteristics of each zone are well illustrated by events following stapling of the LGP.[52] Cartilage cells continue to multiply until pressure builds within the matrix and slows cell proliferation. The cells of the zone of cartilage transformation continue their normal maturation process. The matrix calcifies, the cartilage cells enlarge and degenerate, and metaphyseal vascular loops penetrate to produce bone. In turn, the palisading cells in the zone of growth then mature. Finally the thin layer of reserve cartilage cells adjacent to the bony end plate is replaced by bone, and the metaphysis fuses with the epiphysis. Normal recovery occurs if the staple is removed before all of the growth cartilage cells have been exhausted. It is probably that the plate closes after adolescence by a similar mechanism, namely sequential retrograde depletion of the plate, the proliferating cells of which are not being replenished because of decreasing hormonal stimulus.

Clinical summary

Irreparable injury to proliferating cartilage cells in the *zone of growth* or necrosis as a result of loss of vascularity may result in failure of growth. The remaining cells in the plate mature in sequence, and epiphysiodesis occurs.

Isolated injury to the *zone of transformation* does not influence cell proliferation and only temporarily retards osteogenesis by failing to elaborate

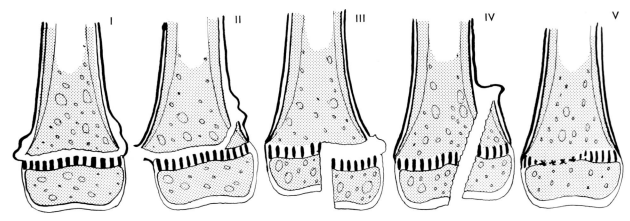

Fig. 5-3. Types of growth plate injury as classified by Salter and Harris. Type I—slipped epiphysis. Type II—slipped epiphysis with a metaphyseal fragment (Thurston-Holland sign). Type III—fracture through the epiphysis, with or without slip of the fragment. Type IV—longitudinal fracture extending through the epiphysis and across the growth plate into the metaphysis. Type V—compression injury causing disruption of the growth plate without roentgenographically demonstrable fracture. (From Rang, M.: Children's fractures, Philadelphia, 1974, J. B. Lippincott Co.)

calcified cartilage matrix as a template for bone formation.

Interruption of bone formation within the *zone of ossification* temporarily inhibits elaboration of primary spongiosa in the metaphysis but does not affect cartilage cell proliferation or transformation.

INJURIES TO THE GROWTH PLATE

In 1898 Poland[42] recognized the difference between epiphyseal slips and epiphyseal fractures that cross the growth plate. Harris[27] differentiated between horizontal growth plate fractures and longitudinal fractures, emphasizing the poor prognosis in the latter. Aitken's[3] concept, much like Poland's, pointed to the poor prognosis of longitudinal fractures across the plate. Salter and Harris[49] developed a classification that remains as the classical guide for prognosis and management of these injuries (Fig. 5-3).

Type I

The zone of cell hypertrophy is the weakest segment of the longitudinal growth plate and the zone where horizontal fractures (slipped epiphysis) occur most frequently. A fall on the outstretched hand, which produces a Colles fracture in an adult, may separate the distal radial epiphysis in a child. Ligaments are attached to the epiphysis, and the impact of injury is transmitted to the adjacent LGP. A lateral force to the knee, for example, which might result in ligament tear, tibial condyle fracture, or avulsion fracture in an adult, more commonly causes slipping of the distal femoral epiphysis in a child. Tenderness above the femoral condyle, even in the presence of a normal roentgenogram, demands stress testing to determine whether a spontaneously reduced slipped distal femoral epiphysis occurred. Since rapid growth and remodeling take place at the ends of bone, a greater degree of angulation is acceptable in slipped epiphyses or metaphyseal fractures than in diaphyseal fractures. As a general guide, Blount[9] established the principle that angulation in the plane of a neighboring ginglymus joint, namely flexion and extension, has greater potential for correction than medial and lateral angulation and that 30 degrees of angulation near the growth plate at age 6 or 7 is acceptable because of the potential for remodeling in that area.

Although the majority of simple Type I frac-tures heal without deformity, recent experience has indicated that epiphysiodesis may occasionally occur. Experimentally, it has been demonstrated[12] that the forces producing a slip may cause ragged disruption of the plate that extends above and below the zone of hypertrophied cells and occasionally into the zone of growth. Anatomically, the growth plate itself may not be completely horizontal, most notably at the distal femur where the plate generally rises in the center corresponding to the intercondylar notch. A fracture line extending transversely across the plate may fracture through hillocks of bone and lead to epiphysiodesis.

The blood supply to the growth plate is derived from vessels that enter the epiphysis directly, close to capsular and ligamentous attachments. Consequently, in a Type I injury, vascularity is rarely compromised. A unique exception is the proximal femoral epiphysis where vessels to the head course through the growth cartilage that surrounds the LGP and extends down onto the neck of the femur. Slipping of the epiphysis, therefore, may disrupt these vessels and lead to avascular necrosis of the bony centrum and the longitudinal growth plate.

Type II

As an epiphysis is displaced, it may carry with it a segment of metaphyseal bone (Thurston-Holland sign). Brashear[10] demonstrated experimentally that a shear force consisting of a combination of lateral thrust and weight bearing may result in a Type II injury as opposed to more of an avulsion component in Type I. The greater forces usually associated with a Type II fracture may increase the risk of LGP damage and traumatic epiphysiodesis.

Type I and Type II injuries usually present little problem in reduction and stability because the periosteum on the side of the displacement is generally intact. In unusual instances of instability, a single or several unthreaded wires across the plate do not jeopardize future growth.[52] When the wires are removed, the channel that remains is not unlike a Type IV injury in that it soon becomes filled with a plug of bone, forming an anatomic epiphysiodesis. Since the amount of growth cartilage that is bridged by a channel formed by a wire is relatively minimal compared with the large unaffected volume of normal growth cartilage, the bony bridge rapidly attenuates under the traction force of growth and becomes replaced by cartilage, generally having no effect on longitudinal growth. Mechanically, one or several smooth thin rigid wires are sufficient to fix the epiphysis to the metaphysis and prevent redisplacement. It is recommended that fixation wires be unthreaded, small in size, and centrally located to avoid the perichondral ring and prevent eccentric effects of epiphysiodesis.

Type III

Type III injury, caused by an intra-articular shearing force, produces a longitudinal fracture through the epiphysis and a slip of the growth plate as the epiphyseal fragment is displaced. Only occasionally does the fracture line continue into the metaphysis as a Thurston-Holland–like fragment (triplane fracture).

Since the fracture line is intra-articular, accurate reduction is essential to avoid irregularity of the joint surface. If open reduction is necessary, fixation can best be accomplished by use of an intraepiphyseal compression screw. In a displaced Type III fracture, a gap between the fragments represents a potential isthmus into which bone from the epiphysis may grow and join metaphyseal bone to form an epiphysiodesis if there is a break in continuity of the reserve and proliferating cartilage cell layer.

Type III fractures occur most commonly at the upper and lower tibia during early adolescence. Normally the growth plate appears to begin its closure eccentrically, thereby protecting a segment of the plate from Type I or Type II injury.

A Type III fracture is generally a consequence of vulnerability of the open portion of the plate, which may be displaced with its adjacent epiphyseal segment. If traumatic epiphysiodesis occurs in Type III injuries close to the time of plate closure, little or no deformity will result. Regardless of age, a displaced fragment should always be reduced, open or closed, to assure integrity of the joint surface.

Occasionally a Type III fracture may occur in a younger child with considerable growth remaining. Unless accurate closed reduction can be accomplished, it is generally advisable to align the fragments and close the gap by use of an intra-epiphyseal compression screw. Care should be taken to place the screw in the safe area[59] in the center of the epiphysis, since the vascular channels that supply the growth plate lie close to the bony end plate.

Type IV

Type IV injury is a longitudinal fracture that extends from the joint surface across the epiphysis and growth plate and into the metaphysis. It represents the highest risk of all fractures because it exposes a channel across the plate into which bridging bone may grow from both the epiphysis and the metaphysis during reparative osteogenesis (Fig. 5-2, *C*). Roentgenographic evidence of separation between fragments signifies a poor prognosis, and even hairline infractions that may not be readily visible on the initial roentgenogram may result in epiphysiodesis.

Accurate reduction can be assured only by

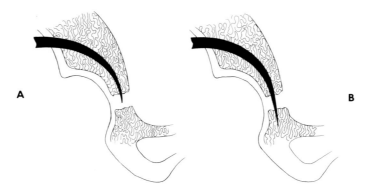

Fig. 5-4. A, Acetabuloplasty procedures that enter the triradiate growth cartilage from the ilium do not result in epiphysiodesis. **B,** If a channel is opened from the ilium to the ischium or pubis by violation of the triradiate cartilage either by osteotomy, excessive intrapelvic periosteal stripping or acetabular rotational procedures in a young child, epiphysiodesis may occur. (From Siffert, R. S.: Skeletal Radiology, **2:**21, 1977.)

opening the joint and meticulously aligning the articular surface. A compression screw through the two fragments of the epiphysis and another through the metaphysis may prevent epiphysiodesis.

Much like a Type IV fracture that crosses growth cartilage, violation of the triradiate cartilage in acetabuloplasty procedures may lead to fusion of the adjacent ilium, ischium, and pubis (Fig. 5-4). A Pemberton osteotomy carried too far across the cartilage into one of the adjacent bones, excessive intrapelvic periosteal stripping that extends across the triradiate cartilage to the ischium or pubis in an innominate or Chiari procedure, or an acetabular rotational osteotomy in a young child may result in triradiate epiphysiodesis. Normally, as appositional cartilage forms on the surface of the acetabulum, the cup-shaped contour of the joint is maintained by interstitial growth of the triradiate cartilage.[43] Epiphysiodesis results in a deformed, small, and shallow acetabulum.[26]

Type V

Type V injury implies a crushing of the plate and generally is a diagnosis made in retrospect. Progressive angulation of an extremity or shortening 6 to 12 months after soft tissue injury or fracture of a long bone, or even without a history of major trauma in an active preadolescent or adolescent may indicate eccentric or central epiphysiodesis in spite of apparently normal initial roentgenograms. Severe crush injury to the LGP leading to epiphysiodesis has been reported,[35,57] but the mechanism of growth arrest in Type V involvement has not been clarified as to whether it is direct crush, vascular damage, unrecognized central fracture through cancellous bone, or all three. It is wise, therefore, in all major injuries to an extremity during the growth period to reexamine the patient 6 months later and to inform parents of the possibility of damage to the growth plate, instructing them how to observe the extremity for angulation or apparent shortening.

In the absence of increasing angulation, early epiphysiodesis may be difficult to recognize. Epiphysiodesis that occurs in the intramedullary section of the plate produces a "tenting" shadow on the roentgenogram (Fig. 5-10, *A*). If centrally located, it may cause slowing of growth, but if eccentric or peripheral may result in angulation. Tomograms are valuable in identifying the exact location and extent of both central and peripheral epiphysiodeses. Prognosis regarding potential deformity depends largely upon age of the patient and future projected growth.

GROWTH ARREST LINES

One of the most valuable indicators of normal or abnormal bone growth following fracture or epiphyseal injury is the growth arrest line. The pathophysiology of growth arrest lines due to trauma probably bears similarities to that resulting from malnutrition.[40] Trauma, perhaps mediated through its metabolic effects on the body as a whole, appears to temporarily inhibit growth cartilage proliferation. As cells of the zone of transformation mature and degenerate, new bone continues to form on available calcified cartilage remnants. In both trauma and malnutrition, when chondrogenesis is slowed, the plate narrows, and a plaque of bone accumulates on calcified cartilage remnants on its metaphyseal surface. When growth resumes, the bone plaque thickens and remains as a growth arrest line and a marker of the date of injury (Fig. 5-5). Growth arrest lines do not occur universally, and therefore their absence cannot always be interpreted as an indication that growth has stopped. Nor do they occur in all bones. The lines are more common in larger bones, notably the tibia and femur, possibly because of summation of many small areas of thickened trabeculae within the metaphysis. Generally they are visible bilaterally, but may be observed unilaterally, occasionally even on the side opposite the bone that had been fractured, indicating that the process is a systemic response to trauma rather than purely a locally induced phenomenon.

Failure of formation of a growth arrest line in the tibia following epiphyseal injury, for example, in the presence of lines in the femur bilaterally and the opposite tibia generally indicates total epiphysiodesis. Partial epiphysiodesis can be identified by a metaphyseal line that is angulated away from the growth plate at the point of growth arrest. When epiphysiodesis is peripheral, a wedge-shaped area of new bone appears between the growth arrest line and the growth plate, indicating the rate of increasing deformity. Identification of the location of epiphysiodesis permits early correction of deformity. A growth arrest line may appear after trauma as a dense line beneath new subchondral bone within the epiphy-

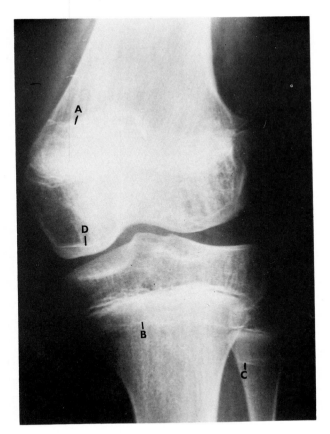

Fig. 5-5. Growth arrest lines represent clinically important markers of posttraumatic growth dynamics. Growth arrest lines appeared horizontally across the distal femur *(A)*, proximal tibia *(B)*, and proximal fibula *(C)* in this 11-year-old boy who sustained a Type V lateral epiphysiodesis of the distal femur. The epiphysiodesis produced complete lateral arrest of growth as indicated by the growth arrest line in the femur. Abnormal pressure effects at the knee subsequently slowed proximal medial tibial growth as indicated by a small amount of new bone that formed above the growth arrest line, while the lateral aspect of the tibia continued to grow almost normally as measured against the growth arrest line in the fibula. A growth arrest line in the epiphysis *(D)* is seen as a dense subchondral condensation, and subsequent epiphyseal cartilage growth can be measured from the growth arrest line to the joint surface.

sis, giving the appearance of a "bone within a bone" (Fig. 5-5).

INJURY TO THE EPIPHYSIS
Articular growth cartilage

Damage to proliferating cells on the surface of an epiphysis may result in irregularity of the surface or in the shape of the epiphysis itself.[38] Cor-rection of the etiologic biomechanical factor during childhood or adolescence, as in recurrent dislocating patella with chondromalacia or humeral condylitis (pitcher's elbow), often permits regeneration of growth cartilage cells. Severe and persistent injury of the cartilage may result in permanent osteochondral and articular surface irregularities. Details regarding the physiology of healing of cartilage defects in children and the longevity of reparative fibrocartilage have yet to be clarified.

Injuries to cartilage and bone

Acute osteochondral fractures include separation of a segment containing bone and overlying cartilage. Accurate closed or open reduction, often with internal fixation, may permit bone healing to occur. The outer layer of cartilage cells that obtain nutrition from the joint surface may remain alive.[36] Although there is experimental evidence of early cartilage reparative responses, completely normal cartilage healing does not appear to occur.[38] The younger the child, the greater the chance that appositional proliferation of surface cartilage cells will cover the fracture defect.

Traumatic osteochondrosis dissecans probably represents a similar type of injury in which an acute or stress insult results in fracture and separation of a fragment of subchondral epiphyseal bone. The overlying cartilage, being resilient, may remain intact, but the underlying avascular bony fragment may not heal.[1,2,31,61] A fibrous barrier between the fragment and epiphyseal bone nucleus, producing a nonunion, may develop, and eventually the bony fragment may absorb. The overlying articular and growth cartilage then being deprived of a mechanical base that is necessary for nutritional diffusion may fracture, degenerate, separate, or become a loose body in the joint. In a young child, early diagnosis and protection by rest and immobilization often permit bone healing, and if a defect exists in the joint surface, it apparently becomes covered by articular proliferating growth cartilage. Satisfactory results have been described as a result of surgical procedures to immobilize the bony fragment and revascularize it by drilling across the fibrous nonunion or bone grafting.

Injury to the bony epiphysis

Loss of vascular supply that produces avascular necrosis of the epiphyseal centrum may be the re-

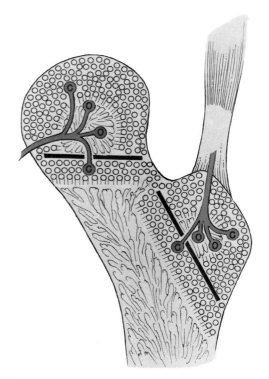

Fig. 5-6. Blood vessels that enter the growing epiphysis and apophysis support both chondrogenesis and osteogenesis by supplying nutrition to the deep portion of growth cartilage, zone of ossification of the bony epiphysis, bone of the epiphysis, and proliferating cells of the longitudinal growth plate. Chondrogenesis, *C;* osteogenesis, *O.*

sult of extraosseous, intraosseous, or idiopathic causes.[55]

Extraosseous loss of vascularity may follow fracture of the neck of the femur,[4] slipped capital femoral epiphysis,[49] surgical or traumatic laceration or thrombosis of the medial or lateral vessels, or infection.

Intraosseous causes may interfere with normal trabecular nutrition and be vascular, as in sickle cell disease, or be metabolic storage effects of Gaucher's disease or steroids. Trauma may be a contributing factor in children who are vulnerable as a result of these conditions.

Idiopathic avascular necrosis, which is known as the Legg-Calvé-Perthes syndrome (LCPS), at the hip is presumed to be at least in part traumatic. Multifactorial elements including immaturity and heredity have been implicated as predispositions.[19,25] On the basis of experimental evidence,

it has been suggested that repeated injuries may be necessary to cause the syndrome.[21,50,67]

The clinical manifestations of idiopathic avascular necrosis in LCPS vary greatly depending partly on the extent of involvement and the age of the patient. Interference with vascular supply to the medial or lateral femoral capital vessels, which supply the femoral head, may produce a variety of changes resulting in widely different clinical findings, depending upon which of the osteogenic and chondrogenic functions are disturbed and to what degree (Fig. 5-7).

Vascular supply to the femoral head during growth supplies nourishment to growth cartilage of the epiphysis and the LGP and bone within the epiphyseal centrum. It is concerned with both osteogenesis and chondrogenesis (Fig. 5-6).

1. Osteogenesis (within in the bony centrum)
   a. New bone formation in the zone of ossification
   b. Maintenance of health of bone within the epiphysis
2. Chondrogenesis
   a. Diffusion of nutrients into the deeper layers of growth cartilage of the epiphysis
   b. Supply of proliferating cells of the longitudinal growth plate by penetrating the bony end plate

Complete avascular necrosis, therefore, as it occurs in LCPS may produce varying degrees of necrosis of the bony centrum depending upon whether the medial and/or lateral vessels are involved. Cessation of osteogenesis and altered chondrogenesis in the epiphysis and destruction of cartilage proliferation at the longitudinal growth plate may result in well-recognized clinical patterns.* Repair always occurs in LCPS as a result of continued appositional growth of the peripheral growth cartilage cells of the epiphysis and eventually revascularization of the epiphysis itself. During this reparative stage, overgrowth of the head, apparently stimulated by hyperemia[51] and subluxation,[55] places the head in an incongruous position in the acetabulum leading to deforming biomechanical effects (Fig. 5-7). Protection of the vulnerable healing femoral head may be obtained by seating it deeply within the acetabulum. This can be accomplished nonsurgically by bracing techniques that place the hip in abduction, or surgically by femoral or innominate osteotomy. In LCPS, segmental avascular necrosis

---

*See references 17, 22, 25, 28, 29, and 55.

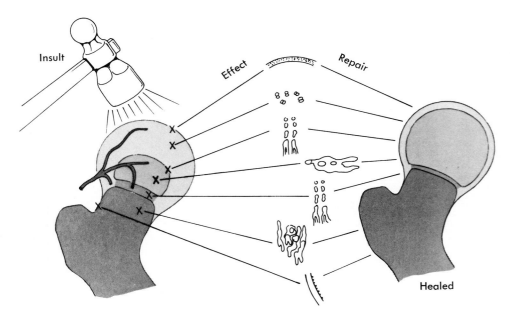

Fig. 5-7. Diagram of the reparative potential of the femoral head in LCPS. Trauma, coupled with constitutional factors, probably represents a major etiologic component. The natural history subsequent to development of necrosis of the bony nucleus depends to a major degree on the location and extent of involvement and to a lesser degree on the method of treatment. Once necrosis has occurred, the following subsequent sequences may take place as growth of articular cartilage continues: disruption of deeper layers of epiphyseal growth cartilage, disruption of osteogenesis of epiphyseal cartilage-bone formation, necrosis of the bony centrum, interruption of blood supply to the LGP, metaphyseal cyst formation, and broadening of the lateral neck. Surgical and nonsurgical techniques that obtain centration of the head within a well-covered acetabulum may minimize the effect of pressure on these reparative mechanisms. (Redrawn from American Academy of Orthopaedic Surgeons: Instructional course lectures, vol. 22, St. Louis, 1973, The C. V. Mosby Co.)

may lead to a syndrome similar to traumatic osteochondrosis dissecans.[31,61] A section of the bony epiphysis and overlying deeper layers of growth cartilage may separate and appear as a free fragment on the roentgenogram. An arthrogram[29] or surgical exploration may reveal that the head outline and surface cartilage, which is nourished by joint fluid, remain intact during the early stage of bony centrum deformity.

The superior and inferior growth plates of a vertebral body may undergo irregular ossification resulting in fragmentation, disc intrusion into the body, separation of the apophyseal ring, and other changes resulting in altered spinal mechanics and progressive structural scoliosis (Scheuermann's disease).[56] The current hypothesis is that these changes probably represent the effects of trauma during adolescence, possibly associated

with as yet undefined aspects of developmental vulnerability. Similarly, trauma of excessive traction forces represents an etiologic factor in disorderly enchondral ossification of the tibial tubercle in Osgood-Schlatter disease.

INJURY TO THE IMMATURE EPIPHYSIS

The Poland,[42] Aitken,[3] Salter and Harris,[49] and other classifications describe trauma to the growth plate under circumstances where there is a bony epiphyseal centrum present and a mature bony end plate. The key to epiphysiodesis and deformity is that injuries resulting in an isthmus across the LCP may lead to bony bridging of epiphyseal-to-metaphyseal bone (Fig. 5-2, *C*).

In the infant and young child, before the epiphyseal centrum has appeared, or is small, and is separated from the metaphysis by a large mass

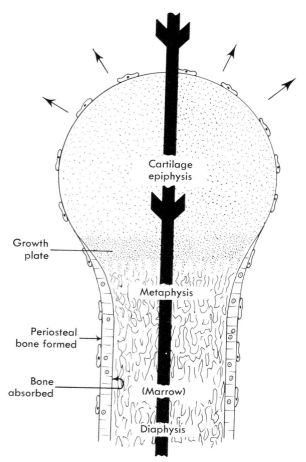

Fig. 5-8. During infancy longitudinal injury across the growth plate from epiphysis to metaphysis does not produce epiphysiodesis, since there is no bone in the epiphysis to join with bone in the metaphysis. If the cartilage center that is destined to form the bony nucleus is divided, two hemicenters will form. (From Siffert, R. S.: Skeletal Radiology **2:**21, 1977.)

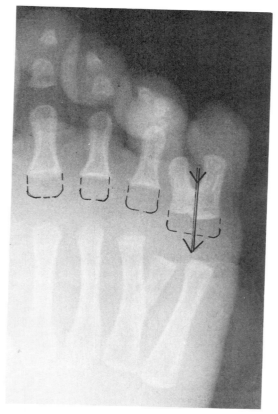

Fig. 5-9. Roentgenogram of the right foot in a 1-year-old infant with six toes. The most lateral proximal phalanx was bifid. Longitudinal bifurcation and amputation of the toe and medial half of the proximal phalanx (and removal of the abnormal fourth lateral metaphyseal segment) was possible without residual epiphysiodesis and deformity by transecting the growth plate before a bony centrum appeared in the epiphysis of the proximal phalanx. (From Siffert, R. S.: Skeletal Radiology **2:**21, 1977.)

of growth cartilage, longitudinal fracture or insults do not result in epiphysiodesis as they do in the older child.[6,45] In infancy and early childhood only Type I fracture (slipped epiphysis) is observed. Type II injury with a Thurston-Holland sign does not occur because of the absence of a bony end plate and resiliency of epiphyseal cartilage to injury. Similarly, Types III, IV, and V fractures through the cartilaginous epiphysis are rarely observed clinically.[45] Theoretically, if they were sustained as a result of injury or produced by surgery, epiphysiodesis would not occur because of absence of epiphyseal bone (Fig. 5-8). This information forms the basis for the evolu-

tion of new principles for reparative and reconstructive surgery in certain congenital abnormalities. It is frequently advisable, for example, to remove a portion of a segmental digit before the bony nucleus appears in order to avoid inevitable epiphysiodesis resulting from performing the procedure when the secondary center of ossification is present (Fig. 5-9). Or the surgery would have to be postponed until full growth of the patient.

Precise bifurcation of a cartilaginous epiphysis through the region where the bony centrum is destined to form will result in the development of two hemicentra at the divided edges. This has

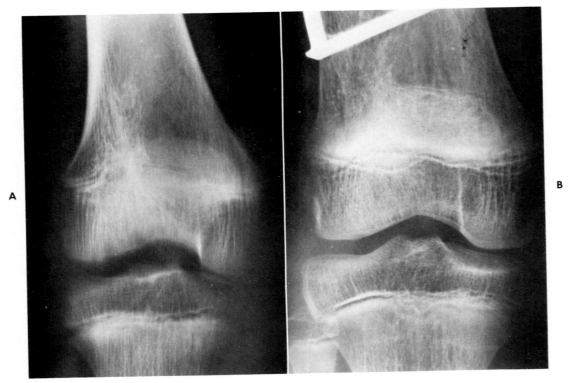

Fig. 5-10. A Type V central "tent" type of epiphysiodesis in a 12-year-old boy with no specific history of injury. **A,** Vertical trabeculae can be identified in this tomogram extending eccentrically from the epiphysis to the metaphysis. **B,** Eighteen months following a corrective osteotomy performed in the metaphysis using internal fixation, the epiphysiodesis has broken away, and longitudinal growth has resumed normally. No growth arrest line formed in the femur probably because of the metaphyseal osteotomy, but the length of time since surgery can be measured by the tibial growth arrest line.

been demonstrated both experimentally[6] and clinically following patella-splitting tenoplasty for congenital dislocation of the knee in Larsen's syndrome.[56]

Except in floppy newborn infants with excessively lax ligaments, an unstable shoulder or elbow joint probably signifies a slipped epiphysis rather than a dislocation. At the elbow,[53] maintenance of the normal olecranon and epicondylar relationships differentiates the injury as a slip of the distal humeral epiphysis rather than a dislocation of the elbow. Slipped upper femoral capital epiphysis[46] may occur following a difficult delivery or in a child who is battered. Rang,[45] summarizing clinical experiences with traumatic epiphyseal fractures, emphasized the difference between nondeforming condylar fractures of the distal humerus through the unossified epiphysis from those through the bony centrum that often result in epiphysiodesis.

CLINICAL MANAGEMENT OF POSTTRAUMATIC EPIPHYSIODESIS

Early recognition of total growth arrest or deformity resulting from eccentric growth plate injuries produced by partial epiphysiodesis permits the orthopaedic surgeon the best opportunity to evolve a rational management regimen to minimize angular deformity or leg length inequality.

If growth retardation or cessation can be identified before gross deformity occurs, a number of treatment alternatives are possible. A growth arrest line,[40,56] when it occurs, is a valuable guide to the early dynamics of deformity.

Epiphysiodesis

When bony angulation occurs as a result of eccentric traumatic epiphysiodesis, surgical obliteration of the remainder of the LGP will halt further progress. Osteotomy may be required to correct deformity that has already occurred, and epiphysiodesis of the contralateral growth plate may minimize leg length inequality. In young children or adolescents of short stature, lengthening of the injured extremity should be considered as an alternative[65] when performance of elective surgical epiphyseodesis of the uninvolved extremity might result in excessive shortening.

Resection of a traumatic epiphysiodesis

Careful identification of the precise site and extent of an epiphysiodesis by tomography facilitates planning of the surgical approach. Bridging bone is meticulously removed by use of a dental burr, leaving an overhanging ledge of growth plate separating the slightly undercut epiphysis and metaphysis. The problem then is to prevent regrowth of bone and reformation of the deformity. Following are procedures that may prevent these two problems:

1. The defect may be packed with autogenous fat.[34,39]
2. Silicone rubber may be pressed into the intertrabecular spaces of the epiphysis and metaphysis to serve as a barrier against new bone formation.[11]
3. Silastic sheeting lining the bone surfaces may be held in place with methyl methacrylate.[41]

Preliminary reports of these relatively new techniques have described some degree of short-term success in preventing recurrence of the epiphysiodesis. Further observations are required to determine the ideal interposition material, the potential for continued clinical long-term growth, and the capability of the plate itself to regenerate without recurrence of deformity.

Following osteotomy to correct angular deformities in Type V injuries, Langenskiold[32] noted resumption of normal longitudinal growth. We have confirmed this observation clinically and have noted that the osteotomy was successful only when the epiphysiodesis was of the central "tent" type (Fig. 5-10) and unsuccessful in Type IV where the epiphysiodesis extended completely across the plate. A theoretic explanation may be that hyperemia, induced by the osteotomy, produces both thinning and osteoporosis of the central cancellous bridge and at the same time stimulates increased cartilage proliferation in the LGP.

SUMMARY

Management of problems associated with premature growth plate closure and leg length inequality[60] demands careful assessment of future growth potential, familiarity with techniques of performing and resecting epiphysiodesis,[11,34,39,41] osteotomy, leg shortening,[8] leg lengthening,[18,65] and evaluation of realistic patient goals. Each child presents an individual problem, and the appropriate selection of surgical techniques depends upon age, height, growth patterns and hereditary, constitutional, and metabolic factors, as well as life-style considerations.

A program designed to prevent epiphyseal injuries is more realistic than treatment once deformity has occurred. Essential ingredients include parental guidance and selection of the right sport and team position for the height, weight, agility, motivation, and skills of a child, coupled with protective equipment, adherence to rules in safe playing areas, professional supervision, training, conditioning, and on-the-spot availability of expert emergency medical care.

REFERENCES

1. Aichroth, P.: Osteochondritis dissecans of the knee, J. Bone Joint Surg. **53-B:**440, 1971.
2. Aichroth, P.: Osteochondral fractures and their relationship to osteochondritis dissecans of the knee, J. Bone Joint Surg. **53-B:**448, 1971.
3. Aitken, A. P.: Fracture of the epiphysis, Clin. Orthop. **41:**19, 1965.
4. Allende, G., and Lezama, L.: Fractures of the neck of the femur in children, J. Bone Joint Surg. **33-A:**387, 1951.
5. Arkin, A. M., and Katz, J. F.: The effect of pressure on epiphyseal growth, J. Bone Joint Surg. **38-A:**1056, 1956.
6. Barash, E. S., and Siffert, R. S.: The potential for growth of experimentally produced hemiepiphyses, J. Bone Joint Surg. **48-A:**1548, 1966.
7. Bentley, G., and Greer, R. B.: The fate of chondrocytes in endochondral ossification in the rabbit, J. Bone Joint Surg. **52-B;**571, 1970.
8. Bianco, A. J.: Femoral shortening, Clin. Orthop. **136:**49, 1978.
9. Blount, W. P.: Fractures in children, Baltimore, 1955, The Williams & Wilkins Co.
10. Brashear, H. R., Jr.: Epiphyseal fractures. A microscopic study of the healing process in rats, J. Bone Joint Surg. **41-A:**1055, 1959.
11. Bright, R. W.: Surgical correction of partial epiphyseal plate closure in dogs by bone bridge resection and use of silicone rubber implants, J. Bone Joint Surg. **54-A:**1133, 1972.
12. Bright, R. W., Burstein, A. H., and Elmore, S. E.: Epiphyseal plate cartilage. A biomechanical and histological analysis of failure modes, J. Bone Joint Surg. **56-A:**688, 1974.
13. Brighton, C. T.: Clinical problems in epiphyseal plate growth and development. In American Academy of Or-

thopaedic Surgeons: Instructional course lectures, vol. 23, St. Louis, 1974, The C. V. Mosby Co., p. 105.

14. Brighton, C. T., and Heppenstall, P. B.: Oxygen tension in zones of the epiphyseal plate, J. Bone Joint Surg. **53-A**:719, 1971.

15. Brower, T. D., Akahoshi, Y., and Orlic, P.: The diffusion of dyes through articular cartilage in vivo, J. Bone Joint Surg. **44-A**:456, 1962.

16. Campbell, C. J., Grisolia, A., and Zanconato, G.: The effects produced in the cartilaginous epiphyseal plate of immature dogs by experimental surgical traumata, J. Bone Joint Surg. **41-A**:1221, 1959.

17. Cattarall, A.: The natural history of Perthes' disease, J. Bone Joint Surg. **53-B**:37, 1971.

18. Coleman, S. S., and Stevens, P. M.: Tibial lengthening, Clin. Orthop. **136**:92, 1978.

19. Duthie, R. B.: The significance of growth in orthopaedic surgery, Clin. Orthop. **14**:7, 1959.

20. Ehrlich, M. G., Mankin, H. J., and Trendwell, B. W.: Biochemical and physiological events during closure of the stapled distal femoral epiphysis in rats, J. Bone Joint Surg. **54-A**:309, 1972.

21. England, J. P. S., and Freeman, M. A. R.: Experimental infarction of the immature canine femoral head, Proc. Soc. Med. **62**:431, 1969.

22. Ferguson, A. B.: The pathology of Legg-Perthes disease and its comparison with aseptic necrosis, Clin. Orthop. **106**:7, 1975.

23. Gardner, E.: Osteogenesis in the human embryo and fetus. In Bourne, G. H., editor: The biochemistry and physiology of bone, vol. 3, ed. 2, New York, 1971, Academic Press Inc., pp. 77-118.

24. Glimcher, M. J., and Krane, S. M.: The organization and structure of bone and the mechanism of calcification. In Gould, B. S., and Ramachandran, G. N., editors: Treatise on collage, vol. 2b, New York, 1968, Academic Press, Inc.

25. Goff, C. W.: Legg-Calvé-Perthes syndrome and related osteochondroses of youth, Springfield, Ill., 1954, Charles C Thomas, Publisher.

26. Hallel, T., and Salvati, E. A.: Premature closure of the triradiate cartilage, Clin. Orthop. **124**:278, 1977.

27. Harris, W. R.: Epiphyseal injuries. In American Academy of Orthopaedic Surgeons: Instructional course lectures, Ann Arbor, Mich., 1958, J. W. Edwards, pp. 15, 206.

28. Jonsater, S.: Coxa plana, Acta Orthop. Scand. (Suppl) **12**:1, 1953.

29. Katz, J. F.: Arthrography in Legg-Calve-Perthes disease, J. Bone Joint Surg. **50-A**:467, 1968.

30. Kuhlman, R. E.: A microchemical study of the developing epiphyseal plate, J. Bone Joint Surg. **42-A**:457, 1965.

31. Lampe, C. E.: Osteochondritis dissecans of the head of the femur, Acta Orthop. Scand. **26**:33, 1957.

32. Langenskiold, A.: The possibilities of eliminating premature partial closure of an epiphyseal plate caused by trauma or disease, Acta Orthop. Scand. **38**:267, 1967.

33. Langenskiold, A.: Premature closure of the distal tibial epiphyseal plate, Acta Orthop. Scand. **38**:520, 1967.

34. Langenskiold, A.: Operative treatment for growth disturbance after epiphyseal injury, Acta Orthop. Scand. **45**:981, 1974.

35. Mankin, H. J.: Localization of tritiated thymidine in artic-

ular cartilage of rabbits, J. Bone Joint Surg. **44-A**:682, 1962.

36. McKibbin, B., and Holdsworth, F. W.: The nutrition of immature joint cartilage in the lamb, J. Bone Joint Surg. **48-B**:793, 1966.

37. McLean, F. C., and Urist, M. R.: Bone. An introduction to the physiology of skeletal tissue, Chicago, 1961, University of Chicago Press.

38. Meachim, G.: The effect of scarification on articular cartilage in the rabbit, J. Bone Joint Surg. **45-B**:150, 1963.

39. Osterman, K.: Operative elimination of partial premature epiphyseal closure, Acta Orthop. Scand. (Suppl), vol. 147, 1972.

40. Park, E. A.: The imprinting of nutritional disturbances on the growing bone, Pediatrics (Suppl) **33**:815, 1964.

41. Peterson, H., and Bianco, A.: Personal communication, 1976.

42. Poland, J.: Traumatic separation of the epiphysis. In Rang, M.: Children's fractures, Philadelphia, 1974, J. B. Lippincott Co.

43. Ponseti, I. V.: Growth and development of the acetabulum in the normal child, J. Bone Joint Surg. **60-A**:575, 1978.

44. Rang, M.: The growth plate and its disorders, Baltimore, 1969, The Williams & Wilkins Co.

45. Rang, M.: Children's fractures, Philadelphia, 1974, J. B. Lippincott Co.

46. Ratliff, A. H. C.: Traumatic separation of the upper femoral epiphysis in young children, J. Bone Joint Surg. **50-B**:757, 1968.

47. Salter, R. B.: Experimental and clinical aspects of Perthes' disease, J. Bone Joint Surg. **48-B**:393, 1966.

48. Salter, R. B., and Field, P.: The effects of continuous compression on living articular cartilage, J. Bone Joint Surg. **42-A**:31, 1960.

49. Salter, R. B., and Harris, W. R.: Injuries involving the epiphyseal plate, J. Bone Joint Surg. **45-A**:587, 1963.

50. Sanchis, M., Zahir, A., and Freeman, M. A. R.: The experimental simulation of Perthes' disease by consecutive interruptions of the blood supply to the capital femoral epiphysis in the puppy, J. Bone Joint Surg. **55-A**:335, 1973.

51. Schiller, M. G., and Axer, A.: Hypertrophy of the femoral head in Legg-Calve-Perthes syndrome, Acta Orthop. Scand. **43**:45, 1972.

52. Siffert, R. S.: The effect of staples and longitudinal wires on epiphyseal growth. An experimental study. J. Bone Joint Surg. **38-A**:1077, 1956.

53. Siffert, R. S.: Displacement of the distal humeral epiphysis in the newborn infant, J. Bone Joint Surg. **45-A**:165, 1963.

54. Siffert, R. S.: The growth plate and its affections, J. Bone Joint Surg. **48-A**:546, 1966.

55. Siffert, R. S.: Osteochondrosis of the proximal femoral epiphysis. In American Academy of Orthopaedic Surgeons: Instructional course lectures, St. Louis, 1973, The C. V. Mosby, p. 270.

56. Siffert, R. S.: The effect of trauma on the epiphysis and growth plate, Skeletal Radiology **2**:21, 1977.

57. Siffert, R. S., and Arkin, A. M.: Posttraumatic aseptic necrosis of the distal tibial epiphysis, J. Bone Joint Surg. **32-A**:691, 1950.

58. Siffert, R. S., and Gilbert, M. S.: Anatomy and physiology of the growth plate, In Rang, M.: The growth plate and its disorders, Baltimore, 1969, The Williams & Wilkins Co., p. 1.

59. Siffert, R. S., and Katz, J. F.: Experimental intraepiphyseal osteotomy, Clin. Orthop, **82:**234, 1972.

60. Stephens, D. C., Herrick, B. S., and MacEwen, G. D.: Epiphysiodesis for limb length unequality. Results and indications, Clin. Orthop. **136:**41, 1978.

61. Stillman, B. C.: Osteochondritis dissecans and coxa plana, J. Bone Joint Surg. **48-B:**64, 1966.

62. Trias, A.: The effect of persistent pressure on the articular cartilage, J. Bone Joint Surg. **43-B:**376, 1961.

63. Trueta, J.: The normal vascular anatomy of the human femoral head during growth, J. Bone Joint Surg. **39-B:**358, 1957.

64. Urist, M. R.: Growth hormone and skeletal tissue metabolism. In Bourne, G. H., editor: The biochemistry and physiology of bone, vol. 2, ed. 2, New York, 1972, Academic Press, Inc.

65. Wagner, H.: Operative lengthening of the femur, Clin. Orthop. **136:**125, 1978.

66. Wuthier, R. E.: A zonal analysis of inorganic and organic constituents of the epiphysis during endochondral calcification, Calcif. Tissue Res. **4:**20, 1969.

67. Zahir, A., and Freeman, M. A. R.: Cartilage changes following a single episode of infarction of the capital femoral epiphysis in the dog, J. Bone Joint Surg. **54-A:**125, 1972.

Chapter 6

Slipped capital femoral epiphysis

Part I

An approach to salvage procedures for poor results in slipped capital femoral epiphysis

CARL L. NELSON

One of the challenges in orthopaedic surgery lies in the further management of the young patient with slipped capital femoral epiphysis who, following treatment or nontreatment, has an unsatisfactory result.[5,11] I shall share with you an approach to treatment of this group of patients, which is small in number but poses a continuing problem for the thoughtful surgeon. These patients from the onset of epiphyseal slipping to approximately 21 years of age represent the nucleus of the problem. A patient early in life with the sequelae of slipped epiphysis is not a candidate for short-term answers as a primary choice of treatment. As the patient's age increases to the fourth or fifth decade, however, the decision becomes easier as the patient develops the diagnostic criteria for degenerative arthritis of the hip. These facts aid the surgeon in determining if the patient is then a candidate for commonly used reconstructive surgery of the hip such as total hip replacement arthroplasty. Although reconstructive surgery of the hip such as total hip replacement arthroplasty has been one of the most exciting and rewarding advances in orthopaedics in modern times, one must be cautious in extending the age range for these procedures.

Experience is limited in dealing with these problems in younger individuals who have unsatisfactory results from slipped capital femoral epiphysis, and most of the discussion of treatment is anecdotal. Consequently, the forms of treatment prescribed throughout the world vary widely, and no uniform treatment pattern has evolved, since few data are available for analysis. It has been said that science is driven by imagination and reigned by logic and data; unfortunately imaginative treatment in this instance has been minimally modified by data. Since there are few data available, the following discussion is a review of an approach to these difficult problems with an attempt to focus on standard, time-tested surgical procedures and to discuss related new and developmental procedures.

DIAGNOSES ASSOCIATED WITH FAILURE

The most common findings associated with a poor result of slipped capital femoral epiphysis are avascular necrosis, chondrolysis, early degenerative arthritis, and slipped capital femoral epiphysis with a deformity of 90 degrees. Other less commonly seen problems are due to failure or imperfections in surgical technique as well as associated sepsis and osteomyelitis. All the sequelae of treatment or nontreatment are due to the residual effects of an incongruous, displaced, damaged, or stiffened joint that brings the patient to the surgeon because of continuing pain or limited function. Limited function appears to be a major consideration in this younger group of patients in contradistinction to older patients with hip disease, who usually appear because of pain.

78

TREATMENT CONCEPTS

The foremost concept in treating the poor results of slipped capital femoral epiphysis is to rely on a conservative approach; many patients do not necessarily need surgery and can be managed by using nonoperative means. One should follow the rule that patients who have a poor result should be asked to find their level of performance that is pain-free and accept that degree of limitation. Upon close questioning, patients often reveal that the only time they have significant pain is during sports activity. Patients who complain that they have had all types of treatment and still cannot play basketball are a classic example. These patients should simply be told to stop the activity that aggravates their symptoms. This simple rule should be adhered to consistently, since many patients in this age group feel they must do all things and may attempt to coerce the unwary physician to make them temporarily active at any cost. These patients are often given short-term solutions to long-term problems, the sequelae of which may be disastrous.

It should be re-emphasized that weight reduction, anti-inflammatory medication, bed rest, traction, and heat are modalities that should precede any form of more advanced therapy and often are successful in maintaining a patient until later life when commonly used reconstructive surgical procedures are more appropriate.

UNILATERAL VS. BILATERAL DISEASE

If and when nonoperative treatment has proven to be of no further value and the patient is incapacitated from disease, surgical procedures should be considered. As pointed out by Lipscomb,[8] available treatment plans may be most clearly considered if patients are divided into two groups: those with unilateral disease and those with bilateral disease.

Unilateral disease

In general, the degree of problem that requires consideration for surgery in unilateral disease is one in which there are severe joint changes that mandate relatively ablative surgical procedures. On the other hand, occasionally there are patients with unilateral hip disease as a result of slipped capital femoral epiphysis who have joint changes that are secondary to early degenerative arthritis. In these unusual instances, one must not fail to reconsider intertrochanteric osteotomy

as a worthwhile choice of surgical procedures. Although osteotomy may not provide a lasting good result, this type of delaying procedure often will afford the patient a significant period of relatively pain-free activity that can be followed by further reconstructive surgical procedures.

More commonly, the changes that require further consideration for treatment are not suitably treated by osteotomy. For the young individual with unilateral involvement who has severe destructive changes and needs to be active, arthrodesis appears to be the treatment of choice. More specifically, if the patient is young, active, large, has unilateral disease, and attitudinally is not amenable to instruction, arthrodesis is clearly indicated. Although it would appear obvious, it should be pointed out that a patient who fits this description is not a candidate for joint replacement. Consequently it is far better to provide the patient with a hip which can be used under these adverse conditions that later can be reconstructed with another operative procedure.

Lipscomb[7,8] has pointed out that if this type of patient does not have unacceptable disability and one is sure that the situation cannot be realistically improved by other surgical procedures, one should advise the patient to postpone the arthrodesis until pain and deformity are severe enough to warrant the procedure. He describes patients treated in this manner who have returned 2 to 10 years later, only then requesting arthrodesis. If the patient can postpone the surgery long enough, another type of reconstructive procedure may be indicated for the patient.

Bilateral disease

The patient with bilateral slipped capital femoral epiphysis with a poor result in each hip poses a dilemma, since the surgeon must consider multiple operative procedures and combinations of procedures. Each patient must be considered individually, and the attributes and restrictions of various procedures must be fully discussed with each patient. Only after assessment and discussion can the surgeon and patient arrive at a decision that is logical and sound.

If a patient has bilateral early changes of degenerative arthritis with preserved joint spaces, one may consider bilateral osteotomy; however, this clinical situation seldom exists. More commonly, the problem for the surgeon is the patient with severe pain, limited function, and destroyed hips. Hopefully, the patient would be a less active, smaller individual who is educable; the less amenable to suggestion and the larger and more active the patient, the less the chance of long-term success. Although there are no data for comparison, much can be said for arthrodesis of the more severely involved hip and an arthroplasty of the opposite side.[7] It should be clear, however, that a definitive answer is not available for the younger patient with severe bilateral hip disease. If one decides to use the combination of rigid, durable arthrodesis and mobile, less durable arthroplasty, it is clear that the surgeon must first have a successful arthroplasty prior to arthrodesis of the opposite hip. It would be a sorry situation if one has a failed arthroplasty that must be converted to a fusion if the other hip is already fused.

Although the combination of arthrodesis and arthroplasty is the traditional approach to bilateral hip disease in younger patients, most patients prefer bilateral arthroplasty and try to avoid arthrodesis because of "stiffness." Most patients do not accept arthrodesis as a treatment of choice. It should be pointed out to patients that they will have motion of the limb through flexion of the spine and that the "stiffness" does not mean they cannot flex the limb.

The decision that presently poses the greatest problem is the determination of the type of arthroplasty that should be employed. Unfortunately, there are no long-term data to review; consequently, the ultimate value of the types of arthroplasty being done can only be made by future comparisons. Because of this, it would appear logical to choose the one with the highest rate of success and the longest follow-up and one that will allow other operative alternatives later if failure occurs. The key is to determine which presently used procedures best fit these criteria.

Cup arthroplasty has been a standard procedure that meets two criteria, that is, long-term follow-up and preservation of bone stock that allows other operative alternatives later in life. The problem for most surgeons is the lack of predictability of this surgical procedure in their hands; however, cup arthroplasty may be a logical alternative for some patients when used by specific surgeons.

Total joint replacement arthroplasty is a highly predictable surgical procedure with relatively short-term follow-up, but, of course, bone stock for later procedures is sacrificed. It may be argued that if performed carefully for the proper patient, a good result may last 25 years, and a second total joint replacement can be done at that time. These concepts, however, are not supported by long-term follow-up and are, therefore, conjectural. Furthermore, the activity patterns of younger individuals do not appear conducive to long-term good results with this type of procedure.

Surface replacement arthroplasty is a developmental procedure in which the long-term results are not known. However, it theoretically appears to be a better alternative than total hip replacement arthroplasty. Surface replacement arthroplasty is a method of joint replacement that does not sacrifice the femoral head and neck, thus preserving the physiologic load transfer function of the proximal femur. With weight bearing there is theoretically minimal deformation of the surface of the femoral head because the subchondral trabeculae are oriented at right angles to the joint surface and provide a structure of maximum rigidity. The major advantage of surface replacement arthroplasty is that the joint is replaced without significant sacrifice of bone, while preservation of the head and neck allows restoration of more normal anatomic and biomechanical parameters of hip function. Furthermore, it has the distinct advantage of being applicable to younger patients, since other operative alternatives such as arthrodesis, total hip replacement, or head and neck resection still can be done following this procedure.

Wagner,[10] in studying resurfacing arthroplasty in 426 patients, has suggested that early follow-up studies show as good a clinical result as obtained by total hip replacement arthroplasty. On the other hand, Freeman[4] and Capello[1] point out that many technical problems were encountered early in their series.

Although 4- to 5-year follow-ups of patients who have had a surface replacement arthroplasty are available, it still should be considered as a developmental procedure that is technically demanding and needs further evaluation. On the other hand, it would seem that this operative procedure is a viable alternative that has theoretic advantages.

CHRONIC SLIPPED EPIPHYSIS WITH MARKED DISPLACEMENT

A final problem that should be addressed when discussing salvage procedures for slipped capital femoral epiphysis is the patient who has a severe slip with marked displacement of the femoral head. Patients with this severe roentgenographic feature have a poor prognosis with any form of treatment, and although pinning in situ and subtrochanteric osteotomy have been advocated, the clinical results of these treatments are inadequate. In general, the most reliable measurement of successful treatment of hip disorders in children is a normal roentgenographic appearance. There is little chance of approaching this criterion in a patient with a severe slipped epiphysis through standard operative procedures. If the roentgenographic appearance remains marked by distortion after surgical treatment, the final result is sure to be poor; consequently, other operative alternatives need to be considered for these specific problems.

One suggested form of treatment that has been used is wedge or cuneiform osteotomy of the femoral neck.[2,3,6,11] This procedure has not been used in general because of the known high rate of complication and consequently has been essentially abandoned as a primary form of treatment for moderate and minimal slips. This procedure at the proper state of development offers salvage when other forms of treatment are sure to fail. One must be aware of the exceptionally good roentgenographic and clinical results that occur when the procedure is successfully performed in severe slipped epiphyses. If one chooses this procedure for those patients in which standard operative procedures are sure to fail, it should be clear that the procedure has inherent risks and must be performed with skill and accuracy. The key to successful treatment appears to be gentleness of surgical technique, the use of power tools, changing of the shear stresses from vertical to horizontal, rigid internal fixation, shortening of the femoral neck, removal of hypertrophic bony tissues, protection of the posterior cervical vessels, and splitting incisions in the periosteum.[11] It would appear that this procedure may be successfully used when dealing with severe slips; however, this procedure needs to be performed by an experienced, talented surgeon and should be considered in principle as a salvage procedure for the difficult hip problem.

REFERENCES

1. Capello, W. N., Ireland, P. H., Tramell, T. R., and Eicher, P.: Conservative total hip arthroplasty—a procedure to conserve bone stock, Clin. Orthop. **134:**59, July-Aug., 1978.
2. Compere, C.: Correction of deformity and prevention of avascular necrosis in late cases of slipped femoral epiphysis, J. Bone Joint Surg. **32-A:**351, 1950.
3. Dunn, D. M.: Severe slipped capital femoral epiphysis and open replacement by cervical osteotomy. In The hip, vol. 3, St. Louis, 1975, The C. V. Mosby Co.
4. Freeman, M. A. R., Cameron, H. V., and Brown, G. C.: Cemented double cup arthroplasty of the hip, Clin. Orthop. **134:**45, July-Aug., 1978.
5. Hall, J. E.: The results of treatment of slipped femoral epiphysis, J. Bone Joint Surg. **39-B:**659, 1957.
6. Klein, A., Joplin, R. J., and Reidy, J. A.: Treatment of slipped capital femoral epiphysis, J.A.M.A. **136:**445, 1948.
7. Lipscomb, P. R.: Reconstructive surgery for bilateral hip-joint disease in the adult, J. Bone Joint Surg. **47-A:**1, 1965.
8. Lipscomb, P. R.: Salvage of the poor results of slipped capital femoral epiphysis, Clin. Orthop. **48:**153, Sept.-Oct., 1966.
9. Lipscomb, P. R., and McCaslin, F. E., Jr.: Arthrodesis of the hip, review of 371 cases, J. Bone Joint Surg. **43-A:**923, 1961.
10. Wagner, H.: Surface replacement arthroplasty. In The hip, vol. 6, St. Louis, 1978, The C. V. Mosby Co., pp. 3-39.
11. Wilson, P. D., Jacobs, B., and Schecter, L.: Slipped capital femoral epiphysis: an end-result study, J. Bone Joint Surg. **47-A:**1128, 1965.

Part II

Slipped capital femoral epiphysis—natural history and etiology in treatment

RAYMOND T. MORRISSY

It is a common feeling among orthopaedic surgeons that Perthes' disease remains the only serious problem in childhood hip disease, since symptomatic congenital dislocation of the hip can be prevented by careful neonatal examination and slipped capital femoral epiphysis (SCFE) can be easily treated by pinning in situ or osteotomy. In 1963 Joplin[22] called SCFE the "still unsolved hip lesion" because of the frequency with which the diagnosis was delayed and the negative effect this had on the outcome. Actually the problem is more serious than that. We are treating SCFE today as the physician treated pneumonia two centuries ago. SCFE remains the "still unsolved hip lesion" because we do not know its cause; we cannot prevent it; we cannot detect all cases; we cannot prevent its most frequent complication, and our best treatment is inadequate by modern standards.

NATURAL HISTORY

Description of the natural history of a disease is recognized as one of the most essential steps in planning effective treatment. It has been known for several decades that approximately 25% of those cases diagnosed as symptomatic SCFE will be bilateral at least on roentgenographic examination. However, in 1953 Klein et al.[24] noted that after several years an additional 21% of those unilateral symptomatic cases of SCFE had developed roentgenographic evidence of a slip on the opposite side. This slip was characterized by being mild in degree and asymptomatic. In 1959, Billings and Severin,[2] using complex roentgenographic positions and measurements to unmask remodeling, estimated the incidence of bilaterality to be 80%. What is still unknown is how many patients who are asymptomatic through childhood and their young adult life actually have experienced an asymptomatic and undetected slip in one or both hips.

One important step in learning the natural history of this disease is to determine if these undetected slips remain forever below the clinical horizon. This answer has come to us over the last decade from roentgenographic, clinical, and anatomic studies.

Murray[29] called the roentgenographic appearance of a healed minimal slip the "tilt deformity" and found it in 40% of the cases with osteoarthritis of the hip that he reviewed. Subsequently, Stulberg et al.[41] noted a similar deformity they felt was due to either Perthes' disease or SCFE in 40% of 75 patients without known prior hip disease who were to have total hip replacement. More recently Solomon[38] examined 327 femoral heads removed for osteoarthritis and found anatomic evidence of major pathology (e.g., Perthes' disease or SCFE) in 33% and minimal femoral head tilt in an additional 18%.

Clinical evidence is accumulating that confirms this progression of mild tilt deformity toward osteoarthritis in later life. An exhaustive review by Jerre[21] in 1950 noted that in all categories of treatment or slipping, the results tend to get worse with age, that is, patients in each successive decade reported poorer results regardless of their classification as to type of slip, type of treatment, and x-ray findings. Two recent reports[8,36] have also indicated that although patients in their fifth and sixth decade are still highly functional and not at all incapacitated, there are beginning signs of deteriorating hip joint function and increasing symptoms, even in those patients who have had in situ pinning of a minimal slipped capital femoral epiphysis.

Our current knowledge of the natural history of SCFE is summarized in Fig. 6-1. Many cases that are subclinical and escape our detection emerge suddenly during adolescence as acute SCFE. A far greater number remain subclinical until later life when they emerge as symptomatic osteoarthritis. In addition, many cases that we recognized and treated by in situ pinning during adolescence, but left with mild deformity, apparently will progress to late osteoarthritis.

Therefore, in the past few years, we have learned more of the natural history of this strange disease, and what we have learned is rather disquieting to those of us who felt that SCFE was a disease that we could treat effectively. This knowledge poses at least two important problems. First, we seem to be leaving one of the major causes of osteoarthritis of the hip undetected and untreated. And, second, our mainstay of treatment, pinning in situ, may be only palliative, that is, it prevents further slipping but not late osteoarthritis.

ETIOLOGY

Historically we have never been very successful at curing a disease or preventing its complications until we knew the cause. It remains unlikely that anyone will find a single cause for SCFE. However, as we continue to observe and study this disease, we are identifying many factors that ap-

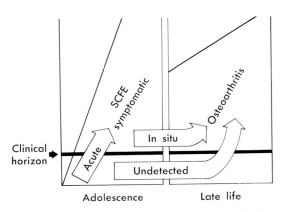

Fig. 6-1. Natural history of slipped capital femoral epiphysis.

pear to be related to its occurrence. These factors are worth mentioning here because some are of clinical importance today, some will probably be important tomorrow, and yet others point the way to future study.

Certain facts of the disease are not disputed. It is a disease of adolescence, a period of altered skeletal development brought about by physiologic hormone changes. It is a disease that is frequently seen in obese children, who are often called Fröhlich. It is a disease occasionally associated with a clinically demonstrable hormone imbalance. All of these factors have been used as circumstantial evidence to support the view that SCFE is caused by a hormone imbalance. Laboratory investigators using animals have focused mainly on the role of growth hormone and estrogen.[3,14,18] They have shown that estrogen increases the strength of the physeal plate, while growth hormone decreases it. The sheer strength of the plate is greater in the female rat than the male, and the strength in both decreases at the time of puberty.

Clinical endocrine investigations to date have failed to provide an explanation for the majority of cases.[34,39] However, it is essential that we keep an open mind to this possibility and understand the technical limitations in measuring hormone levels in vivo accurately under which these investigators worked.

There are a small number of cases that occur with, and seem to be caused by, an endocrine disorder. The most frequently reported are hypothyroidism,[26] hyperparathyroidism,[5] hypogonadal conditions[33] (e.g., cryptorchidism and Klinefelter's syndrome), and panhypopituitarism either before or after substitution therapy.[11,16] Following are clues for the orthopaedic surgeon that will help in the diagnosis of clinical endocrine syndromes associated with SCFE:

Be suspicious if:
  The patient is very tall or very short
  There is sudden or unexpected change in growth
  The patient is under 10 years or over 16 years
Always examine:
  Gonadal size
  Visual fields
Note on radiographs:
  Bone density
  Bone age

Just as there is circumstantial evidence in pointing to a hormone etiology, there is circumstantial

evidence implicating trauma, which may best be understood in this context as the usual muscular and weight-bearing forces generated in everyday activity.

Murray[30] related the incidence of tilt deformity with the amount of athletic activity of the individual during the young, growing years and found that it was directly correlated with the amount of athletic activity. Chung[6] has suggested that it is possible, within the forces that are physiologically generated in the teenage years, to slip the proximal femoral epiphysis. Supporting evidence for this is in the fact that the peak age incidence for all epiphyseal fractures in girls is 11 to 12 years and in boys 13 to 14 years, with boys being affected twice as often; these figures are similar to those for SCFE.[32]

These associations, however, do not answer the whole question. It would indeed be difficult to deny a role to gravity and muscular forces in the slipping of the epiphysis. What is unanswered is whether these forces are the sole factor in causing the slip or if there is some underlying abnormality that allows these normal forces to slip the epiphysis. In other words, is SCFE an accident like a fractured femur, or is it a disease?

Another factor that is associated with SCFE is a familial incidence. When searched for, this familial incidence has been found.[35,42] When one is aware of the likelihood that much of this disease goes undiagnosed, it may be that the familial incidence is even greater. The casual reader should not conclude that this means a hereditary predisposition to the disease. The work of Kelsey et al.[23] showed that incidence of the disease varied significantly in different parts of the country and thus may be due, at least in part, to environmental factors.

Howorth[19] was probably the first to call attention to the synovitis that seems to invariably accompany SCFE. Whether the synovitis is primary or secondary to the slip or what role the synovitis may play in complications is unknown. An interest in the associated synovitis has recently been reawakened by knowledge of the wide-ranging role that the autoimmune system may play in various diseases. In addition, recent reports[10] of increased levels of serum immunoglobulins in patients with SCFE and chondrolysis have heightened interest in the possibility of these being autoimmune diseases.

Our interest in the possible role of synovitis in SCFE was stimulated by two questions that have gone without adequate explanation. The tilt deformity can occur in a hip that was pinned prophylactically.[27] Could this result from the inflammation rather than actual slipping of the epiphysis? The second unexplained question is how does a mild mechanical derangement of the bone produce an inflammation of the synovium?

In an effort to establish answers to these questions, we investigated 15 consecutive cases of SCFE with serum immunoglobulins and synovial biopsies, which were studied with immunofluorescent staining. The results[27,28] have demonstrated that this synovitis is one in which the immune mechanism is active, but what its role may be requires further study.

TREATMENT

Since we are dealing with a disease we cannot prevent and do not know the cause of, our treatment remains empiric, that is, relying or based solely on experiment and observation. While we remain in this situation, we must be very careful in our evaluation of clinical experiments, or more commonly, clinical observations.

About 25 years ago, nonoperative treatment of SCFE was generally abandoned because sufficient evidence had accumulated in the literature to indicate that operative treatment produced better results. Over the past 25 years, our treatment has not changed significantly. Consequently, our results have not changed either. What may be surprising, however, is that even these short-term results have not been very good, with a consistent 20% failure to achieve an acceptable result regardless of the surgeons, the country, the race, etc. (Table 4).

Without a dramatic new cure or a radically different treatment, our only hope of altering these poor results is to examine our current treatment and attempt to improve it. This is not unlike Detroit attempting to get one more mile per gallon from the gasoline engine while waiting for a new technologic breakthrough.

The leading cause of short-term failure is avascular necrosis, with chondrolysis next. Although these complications are not completely under our control, their occurrence can be affected to some degree by factors that we do control. These factors are delay in diagnosis, the amount of displacement when diagnosed, and the type of surgery used.

Table 4. Short-term results of treatment

Author	Date	Satisfactory (%)	Unsatisfactory (%)
Cleveland et al.[7]	1950	80	20
Hall[13]	1957	78	22
Wilson et al.[42]	1965	82	18
Hartman and Gates[15]	1972	80	20

All of these are interrelated. As demonstrated by Jacobs,[20] the amount of displacement is directly related to the delay in diagnosis. He noted that the average duration of symptoms in slight displacement was 13 weeks, in moderate displacement, 24 weeks, and in severe displacement, 40 weeks. He also found that 31% of these patients were subjected to diagnostic error, the major reason being misreading of the roentgenograms and the misleading signs and symptoms of little pain or pain referred to the knee. Therefore, in addition to parent and teacher education (especially physical education teachers and coaches), we need to spend more time educating our primary care colleagues about what to the orthopaedic surgeon is an easy diagnosis.

The amount of displacement has a significant bearing on bad results, as was shown by Jerre,[21] who found 75% good and 5.7% poor results among slight slips and 21.6% good and 32% poor results among severe slips. Various authors have directly related the amount of slipping to avascular necrosis, chondrolysis, and osteoarthritis.

The type of surgery that is done may also have a profound effect on the incidence of complication, especially avascular necrosis. Table 5 compares the incidence of avascular necrosis in various forms of treatment. It is suggested, but not conclusively shown, that the incidence of avascular necrosis in acute slips can be decreased if reduction is achieved by preliminary traction, as opposed to manipulation during anesthesia.[4,37] The incidence of avascular necrosis in those cases which are treated by open reduction or osteotomy of the femoral neck is significant in virtually all series that include a large number of cases, which suggests caution in basing conclusions on one's personal experience. The relationship of treatment to the incidence of chondrolysis is less clear, although its association with subtrochanteric osteotomy has been questioned.[12]

Table 5. Relationship of type of treatment to incidence of avascular necrosis

Author	Treatment	Avascular necrosis (%)
Aadalen et al.[1]	Manipulation during anesthesia with fixation or epiphysiodesis or both	15.0
Hall[13]	Cervical osteotomy	38.1
	Manipulation and nail	37.5
	Nonoperative	12.5
	Manipulation and cast	9.1
	Nail in situ	5.0
	Pins in situ	0.0
Wilson[42]	In situ fixation	0.0
	Trochanteric osteotomy	0.0
	Osteoplasty	0.0
	Manipulation and pin	17.0
	Cervical osteotomy	6.6
Dunn[9]	Open reduction	15.0
Southwick[40]	Intertrochanteric osteotomy	0.0
Herndon[17]	Epiphysiodesis	0.0
	Osteoplasty	0.0

In 1977 O'Brien and Fahey[31] reported on long-term results in a small group of severe slips that were not reduced. They recorded improvements in the range of motion, which would not have been expected, and attributed this to remodeling of the femoral neck. Although other factors may also be responsible, this improvement in the range of motion beyond what would be expected from the residual deformity has been observed in my limited experience and that of others. This calls for a re-evaluation not only of the type of osteotomy, but also of its need and timing.

In summary, we are dealing with a disease, the cause of which usually remains unknown. Therefore, our treatment is empiric and/or imperfect, meaning we must evaluate our results carefully. In so doing, we can identify delayed diagnosis as a major factor in poor results, indicating a need for us to better educate our primary care colleagues. Complications from various forms of treatment are an additional factor that we can control. Thus, we need to evaluate our current surgical procedures and their indications. Most importantly, we must realize that our available treatments are not adequate and continue to search for factors that would enable us to prevent this disease.

REFERENCES

1. Aadalen, R. J., Weiner, D. S., Hoyt, W., and Herndon, C. H.: Acute slipped capital femoral epiphysis, J. Bone Joint Surg. 56-A:1473, 1974.
2. Billing, L., and Severin, E.: Slipping epiphysis of the hip: a roentgenological and clinical study based on a new roentgen technique, Acta Radiol. Suppl. 174, 1959.
3. Bright, R. W., Burstein, A. H., and Elmore, S. M.: Epiphyseal plate cartilage: a biomechanical and histological analysis of failure modes, J. Bone Joint Surg. 56-A:688, 1974.
4. Casey, B. H., Hamilton, H. W., and Bobechko, W. P.: Reduction of acutely slipped upper femoral epiphysis, J. Bone Joint Surg. 54-B:607, 1972.
5. Chiroff, R. T., Sears, K. A., and Slaughter, W. H., III: Slipped capital femoral epiphysis and parathyroid adenoma, a case report, J. Bone Joint Surg. 56-A:1063, 1974.
6. Chung, S. M. K., Batterman, S. C., and Brighton, C. T.: Sheer strength of the human femoral capital epiphyseal plate, J. Bone Joint Surg., 58-A:94, 1976.
7. Cleveland, M., Bosworth, D. M., Daly, J. N., and Hess, W. E.: Study of displaced capital femoral epiphyses, J. Bone Joint Surg. 33-A:955, 1951.
8. Cordell, L. D.: Slipped capital femoral epiphysis: long-term results. Paper presented at the Forty-third Annual Meeting of the American Academy of Orthopaedic Surgeons, New Orleans, February, 1976.
9. Dunn, D. M.: Severe slipped capital femoral epiphysis and open replacement by cervical osteotomy. In The hip, vol. 3, St. Louis, 1975, The C. V. Mosby Co.
10. Eisenstein, A., and Roghschild, S.: Biochemical abnormalities in patients with slipped capital femoral epiphysis and chondrolysis, J. Bone Joint Surg. 58-A:459, 1976.
11. Fidler, M. W., and Brook, C. G. D.: Slipped upper femoral epiphysis following treatment with human growth hormone, J. Bone Joint Surg. 56-A:1719, 1974.
12. Frymoyer, J. W.: Chondrolysis of the hip following Southwick osteotomy for severe slipped capital femoral epiphysis, Clin. Orthop. 99:120, 1974.
13. Hall, J. E.: The results of treatment of slipped femoral epiphysis, J. Bone Joint Surg. 39-B:659, 1957.
14. Harris, W. R.: The endocrine basis for slipping of the upper femoral epiphysis, J. Bone Joint Surg. 32-B:5, 1950.
15. Hartman, J. T., and Gates, D. J.: Recovery from cartilage necrosis following slipped capital femoral epiphysis, Orthop. Rev. 1:33, 1972.
16. Heatley, F. W., Greenwood, R. H., and Boase, D. L.: Slipping of the upper femoral epiphysis in patients with intracranial tumors causing hypopituitarism and chiasmal compression, J. Bone Joint Surg. 58-B:169, 1976.
17. Herndon, C. H., Heyman, C. H., and Bell, D. M.: Treatment of slipped capital femoral epiphysis of epiphyscodesis and osteoplasty of the femoral neck: a report of further experiences, J. Bone Joint Surg. 45-A:999, 1963.
18. Hillman, J. W., Hunter, W. A., Jr., and Barrow, J. A., III: Experimental epiphysiolysis in rats, Surg. Forum 8:566, 1957.
19. Howorth, M. B.: Slipping of the upper femoral epiphysis, J. Bone Joint Surg. 31-A:734, 1949.
20. Jacobs, B.: Diagnosis and natural history of slipped capital femoral epiphysis. In American Academy of Orthopaedic

Surgeons: Instructional course lectures, vol. 21, St. Louis, 1972, The C. V. Mosby Co., p. 167.

21. Jerre, T.: A Study in slipped upper femoral epiphysis, Acta Orthop. Scand. Supp. 6, p. 3, 1950.

22. Joplin, R. J.: Slipped capital femoral epiphysis: the still unknown adolescent hip lesion, J.A.M.A. **188:**379, 1964.

23. Kelsey, J. L., Keggi, K. J., and Southwick, W. O.: The incidence and distribution of slipped capital femoral epiphysis in Connecticut and Southwestern United States, J. Bone Joint Surg. **52-A:**1203, 1970.

24. Klein, A., Joplin, R. J., Reidy, J. A., and Hanelin, J.: Management of the contralateral hip in slipped capital femoral epiphysis, J. Bone Joint Surg. **35-A:**81, 1953.

25. Maurer, R. C.: Acute necrosis of cartilage in slipped capital femoral epiphysis, J. Bone Joint Surg. **52-A:**39, Jan., 1970.

26. Moorefield, W. G., Urbaniak, J. R., Ogden, W. S., and Frank, L. J.: Acquired hypothyroidism and slipped capital femoral epiphysis, J. Bone Joint Surg. **58-A:**705, 1976.

27. Morrissy, R. T.: Slipped capital femoral epiphysis. What's new? In The hip, vol. 6, St. Louis, 1978, The C. V. Mosby Co.

28. Morrissy, R. T., Kalderon, A. E., and Gerdes, M. E.: Autoimmunity in slipped capital femoral epiphysis and chondrolysis. (In Preparation)

29. Murray, R. O.: The aetiology of primary osteoarthritis of the hip, Br. J. Radiol. **38:**810, 1965.

30. Murray, R. O., and Duncan, C.: Athletic activity in adolescence as an etiological factor in degenerative hip disease, J. Bone Joint Surg. **53-B:**406, Aug., 1971.

31. O'Brien, E. T., and Fahey, J. J.: Remodeling of the femoral neck after in situ pinning for slipped capital femoral epiphysis, J. Bone Joint Surg. **59-A:**62, 1977.

32. Peterson, C. A., and Peterson, H. A.: Analysis of the incidence of injuries to the epiphyseal growth plate, J. Trauma **12:**275, 1972.

33. Primiano, G. A., and Hughston, J. C.: Slipped capital femoral epiphysis in a true hypogonadal male (Klinefelter's Mosaic XY/XXY), J. Bone Joint Surg. **53-A:**597, 1971.

34. Razzano, C. D., Nelson, C., and Eversman, J.: Growth hormone levels in slipped capital femoral epiphysis, J. Bone Joint Surg. **54-A**(6):1224, Sept., 1972.

35. Rennie, A. M.: Familial slipped upper femoral epiphysis, J. Bone Joint Surg. **49-B:**535, 1967.

36. Ross, P. M., Lyne, D. E., and Morawa, L. G.: The long-term follow-up of slipped capital femoral epiphysis. Paper presented at the Forty-third Annual Meeting of the American Academy of Orthopaedic Surgeons, New Orleans, February, 1976.

37. Schein, A. J.: Acute severe slipped capital femoral epiphysis, Clin. Orthop. **51:**151, 1967.

38. Solomon, L.: Patterns of osteoarthritis of the hip, J. Bone Joint Surg. **58-B:**196, 1976.

39. Sorensen, H. K.: Slipped upper femoral epiphysis, Acta Orthop. Scand. **39:**499, 1968.

40. Southwick, W. O.: Osteotomy through the lesser trochanter for slipped capital epiphysis, J. Bone Joint Surg. **49-A:**807, 1967.

41. Stulberg, S. D., Cordell, L. D., Harris, W. H., Ramsey, P. L., and MacEwen, G. D.: Unrecognized childhood hip disease: a major cause of idiopathic osteoarthritis of the hip. In The hip, vol. 3, St. Louis, 1975, The C. V. Mosby Co.

42. Wilson, P. D., Jacobs, B., and Schecter, L.: Slipped capital femoral epiphysis: an end-result study, J. Bone Joint Surg. **47-A:**1128, 1965.

Part III

Advantages and disadvantages of pin fixation in slipped capital femoral epiphysis

G. DEAN MacEWEN

INDICATIONS

It is generally agreed that avascular necrosis and cartilage necrosis produce the major problems encountered with slipped capital femoral epiphysis. It is my feeling that pin fixation will help avoid these complications. Indications for multiple pin fixations are (1) a chronic slip with an open epiphyseal line and (2) an acute slip, except where the epiphysis may be completely separated. An acute slip, where the epiphysis is completely separated and will not reduce by traction, is the rare indication for an open reduction. If cartilage necrosis is already present, bed rest is usually recommended and a therapy program is started to regain motion before inserting multiple pins. After the epiphyseal line has closed, an intertrochanteric procedure can be selected to improve the hip joint mechanics. Often, however, with remodeling of the head and neck, no secondary procedure is necessary. Also, there is no proof that changing the mechanics of the joint will delay the onset of osteoarthritis so this should not become the indication for a secondary procedure.

ADVANTAGES

Following are the advantages of pin fixation:
1. The method is relatively simple.
2. There is minimal blood loss because a small lateral incision can be used.
3. One need not open the hip joint, which can be particularly important in the overweight individual where infection is a significant risk.
4. The pins usually can be easily removed after

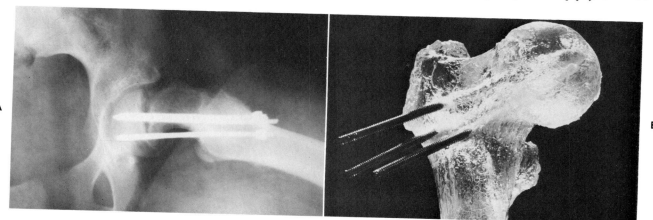

Fig. 6-2. A, Pin placed through lateral cortex exits and re-enters the femoral neck. **B,** Pins enter at base of neck anteriorly and do not penetrate neck posteriorly before entering the femoral head, as shown on plastic model.

the epiphysis is closed if the proper pins are selected.

5. There has been no total avascular necrosis as a result of pin insertion without manipulation.

DISADVANTAGES

One disadvantage of multiple pins is difficulty of insertion in the severe chronic slip. If the pins are placed through the lateral cortex in a severe slip, they must exit through the back of the femoral neck and then re-enter the head (Fig. 6-2, *A*). This allows for the risk of damage to the blood vessels running along the neck. The pins also may penetrate the capsule and thus restrict hip motion. This can also produce problems related to a pin in the joint. However, if the pins are started anteriorly at the base of the neck, just outside the capsule, they can be directed posteriorly, remain in the neck, and engage the femoral head epiphysis (Fig 6-2, *B*). By using this technique, any degree of posterior slip can be stabilized.

Pins can cross the joint surface (Fig. 6-3); therefore, before closure of the wound, two permanent roentgenograms (an anteroposterior and a true lateral or full frogleg view) are necessary to determine if the pins have crossed the epiphyseal line but still are not through the cartilage surface. One should not rely on the image intensification technique as the final view.

Clustering of pins on the weight-bearing surface can produce a segmental avascular necrosis

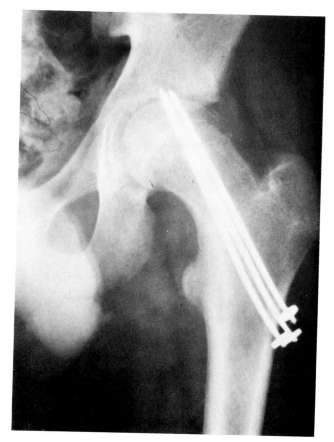

Fig. 6-3. Pins are too long, thus damaging weight-bearing area of acetabulum.

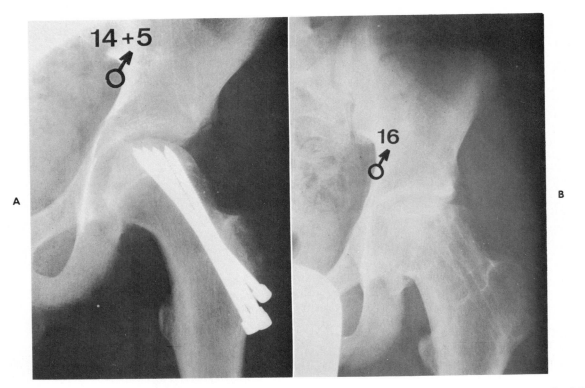

Fig. 6-4. A, Male, 14 years, 5 months of age, had four pins inserted into the subchondral area of the weight-bearing portion of the femoral head without previous manipulation. **B,** Patient in **A** at age 16 after closure of the epiphyseal line and removal of the pins. There has been a segmental avascular collapse of the femoral head directly above the area where the pins were placed.

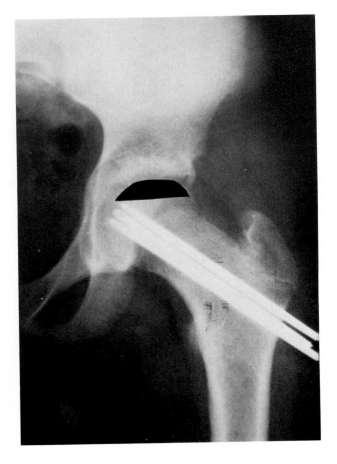

Fig. 6-5. Region to be avoided by the pins is marked in black. Ideal pin placement is shown.

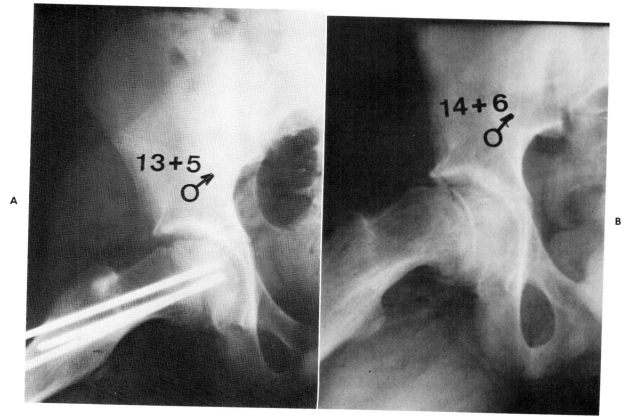

Fig. 6-6. A, Male age 13 years, 5 months, 9 months after pin insertion. Pins were removed prematurely. Note that the epiphyseal line is still open. **B,** Patient in **A,** 13 months later, showing that the epiphyseal line has widened and further slippage has occurred, secondary to premature pin removal.

(Fig. 6-4). The pins should avoid this area. One can mark the roentgenograms before surgery to remind the surgeon to avoid the area (Fig 6-5).

Overreduction of the acute slip must be avoided before the pin is inserted. The acute slip should be reduced by gradual traction, or if reduced with the patient under anesthesia on a fracture table, the force used should be minimal to avoid blood vessel damage.

A complication is the removal of the pin before the epiphyseal line is completely closed, which may lead to further slip. The pins should remain until the epiphyseal line is completely closed (Fig. 6-6 *A*). Even with narrowing of the epiphyseal line, if the pins are removed early, the line can grow again and produce a secondary slip (Fig. 6-6, *B*). At times a planogram may be helpful to determine if the epiphyseal line has completely closed.

Fracture of the shaft can occur after pin re-moval, especially if a large segment of cortex must be removed. The patient should be restricted to walking with a crutch for a few weeks after pin removal to minimize this risk.

It is our belief that, when possible, all pins should be removed after epiphyseal line closure to allow for easier reconstructive surgery later, if this becomes necessary.

TYPES OF PINS

A type of pin that has been used for multiple pinning is the Hagie pin, which is undesirable because the threaded area is larger than the unthreaded base, making it difficult to remove. Even the Gouffon pin, which has a reverse cutting thread, is difficult to remove. The cortical encasement that surrounds the pins after a time makes it almost impossible to remove pins in which the threaded distal end is larger than the unthreaded shaft segment. Pins that are too small

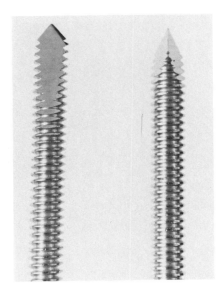

Fig. 6-7. The diamond-tip pin (left) is difficult to remove after bony growth. The trocar pointed pin (right) is much easier to remove.

may fracture, especially if used in an acute slip. Nonthreaded pins generally should not be used because of the risk of migration. The only indication for such pins would seem to be in a very young child with a metabolic problem, who has produced a slip. The use of the pins will keep the epiphysis open and allow time for the metabolic problem, such as hypothyroidism, to be corrected. I prefer threaded ⁹/₆₄ inch Steinmann pins that are cut off outside the cortex at the desired length to allow easy removal later. The full length of the original pin is not critical and thus eliminates one variable. The Knowles pin is ideal, but the length is important, since the cut must be near the lateral cortex. The compression concept across the epiphyseal line does not seem to be important; thus, a threaded pin of constant diameter seems sufficient. The shape of the tip of the pin is also important, for it relates to removal (Fig. 6-7). A flat-sided tip is difficult to extract after the cortical bone has grown around it. A diamond-pointed pin is a little more difficult to insert but allows for easy removal.

SUMMARY

Multiple pin fixation is a satisfactory technique for essentially all patients with an acute or chronic slipped capital femoral epiphysis. However, great attention to detail is necessary to avoid numerous potential complications.

Part IV

Anatomic aspects of slipped capital femoral epiphysis and correction by biplane osteotomy

CHARLES R. CLARK
WAYNE O. SOUTHWICK
JOHN A. OGDEN

Even though advances have been made in our understanding of the patterns of blood supply to the growing capital femoral epiphysis, as well as the possible biomechanics of slipping, treatment for this disease remains relatively unchanged and still somewhat controversial. Since many surgeons find it difficult to carry out corrective operations at a distance from the lesion, they often prefer an intracapsular operation at the deformity itself to achieve a more anatomic correction, while others, considering the extreme danger of direct assault on the injured epiphysis, prefer other alternatives at a safe distance from the critical intracapsular blood supply. Part IV demonstrates some of the newer anatomic physiologic characteristics of this enigmatic disease. It also describes our preferred means of correction and compares it to some other methods in current use.

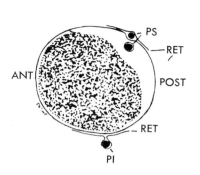
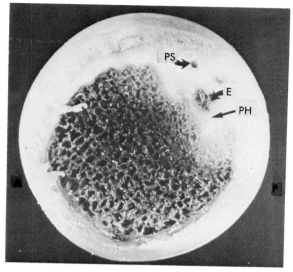

Fig. 6-8. Section of femoral neck in the subcapital region, comparable to the cut performed in a neck osteotomy. The posterosuperior *(PS)* vessels run on or in the cartilage that is always present along this portion of the femoral neck. The posteroinferior *(PI)* vessel tends to be a more mobile retinaculum *(RET)*. *E* signifies a portion of the epiphyseal ossification center (majority of bone is the femoral neck or metaphyseal); *PH* is the physeal cartilage.

BLOOD SUPPLY TO THE GROWING CAPITAL EPIPHYSIS

During the age range susceptible to slipped capital femoral epiphysis, a well-developed femoral neck has appeared, necessitating a significant intracapsular course for the two primary vessels, the posterosuperior and the posteroinferior, supplying the capital femur[13] (Fig. 6-8). The posteroinferior vessel generally is contained within a mobile, retinacular fold and probably is not compromised by a slip. However, this vessel is the secondary blood supply of the capital femoral ossification center. As the capital femur and greater trochanter grow apart from the development of the femoral neck, a bridge of epiphyseal cartilage remains, even in later adolescence, along the posterosuperior neck (Fig. 6-9). The primary blood supply to the capital femoral ossification center, the posterosuperior artery, runs directly along or within this cartilage. As the femoral head slips, this vessel may be attenuated, compromising its ability to adequately vascularize the ossification center. Operative procedures involving the femoral neck must cut across the posterosuperior cartilage bridge, and, in so doing, may totally transect the posterosuperior

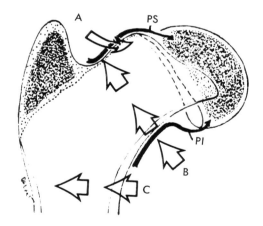

Fig. 6-9. Schematic presentation of the blood supply in slipped capital femoral epiphysis. *PS,* posterosuperior vessels; *PI,* posteroinferior vessels; *A,* acute or chronic slip. The posterosuperior vessel is more likely to be compromised physiologically or morphologically; *B,* osteotomies across the femoral neck, either at the subcapital level or lower, run a significant risk of injuring one or both vessels; *C,* osteotomy at the lesser trochanteric level should not jeopardize the intracapsular vessels.

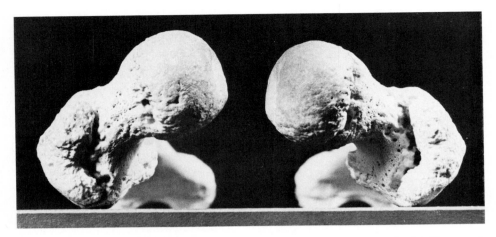

Fig. 6-10. Normal anteversion seen in juvenile hip specimens. Note the highly vascular openings all along the superior neck in both specimens. Note also how pressure on the superior portion of the femoral head epiphysis tends to be in the posterior axis of the femoral head and neck and pushes the head into varus and posterior tilt.

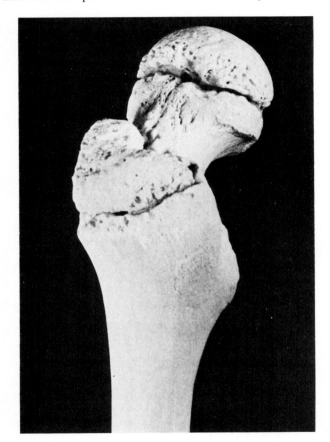

Fig. 6-11. Lateral view of specimen in Fig. 6-10 shows trochanter, trochanteric epiphysis, neck, and capital epiphysis. Note how the capital epiphysis normally tilts posteriorly, just prior to the preadolescent growth spurt.

blood supply (Fig. 6-9). Anastomoses between these two systems exist at the subsynovial level and within the ossification center, but there may not be sufficient flow to allow the posteroinferior system to take over the physiologic function of the posterosuperior system. Operative procedures at the lesser trochanteric level should not disturb the intracapsular vascularity.

MECHANICS OF SLIPPING

There are many theories that attempt to explain why the juvenile femoral head slips through the growth plate in adolescent children. Since this condition occurs only during periods of rapid growth, it is reasonable to believe that during such periods the columnar zone, which is known to be considerably thicker and more fragile, may shear as a result of relatively minor forces. Children who have endocrinopathies or who are grossly overweight seem particularly susceptible.[15] The summation of forces at the joint seems almost invariabley to produce a varus, posterior-tilting deformity of the head of the femur so that the head slips with respect to the neck, giving the patient deformity of external rotation and shortening.

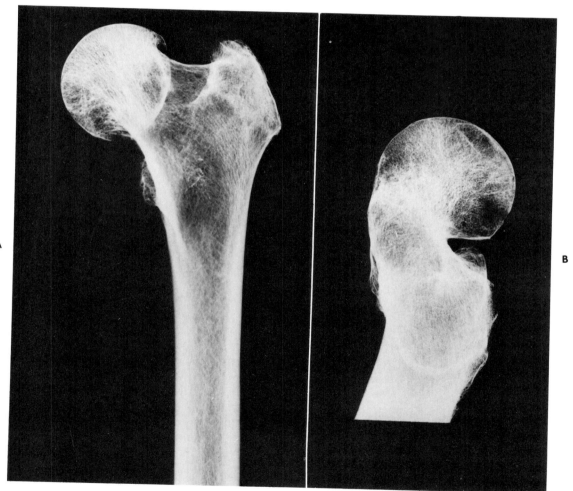

Fig. 6-12. A, Specimen of a femur with slipped capital femoral epiphysis shows the varus and posterior tilt of the head as seen in the AP plane. (Courtesy Dr. Dean Mc-Ewen.) **B,** Lateral view of same specimen. Posterior tilt of the femoral head is clearly visible. The lines of trabeculae have altered to the superior surface of weight bearing. Notice the cystic changes in the area of disuse posteriorly, which would eventually lead to arthritic degeneration.

An anatomic explanation for the most common type of slips is anteversion of the femoral neck (Fig. 6-10) and the relative posterior tilting of the epiphyseal plate of the head of the femur (Fig. 6-11). When the joint reaction force passes from the shaft of the femur through the femoral head to the acetabulum, it would appear to have its greatest pressure on the posterosuperior axis of the head of the femur. If anteversion of the neck and posterior tilt at the epiphyseal plate are subjected to increased tension and shear stresses, the rapidly growing epiphysis may not be sufficiently strong and gives way. As with fractures of this area, forces of external rotation are poorly counteracted, and the femoral neck externally rotates while the head tilts posteriorly on the neck. Posterior tilt should be considered a product of external rotation of the neck (metaphysis) because the head is restrained within the acetabulum by the capsule, the ligamenta capitis femoris, and suction. Whatever the various mechanisms, the net effect is that the vast majority of patients have an external rotation deformity of the femoral shaft, posterior tilt of the head on the posterior neck of the femur, and a varus angulation (Fig. 6-12). The varus angulation is thought of more as a product of shortening. A more accurate method of describing the deformity is to note that the distal fragment, the femoral neck, has displaced into external rotation and shortening. However, tradition dictates the former, describing the head with respect to the neck. The few cases of valgus slip are rare and often are associated with some metabolic disorder such as Marfan's disease.

REVIEW OF TREATMENT METHODS

Manipulation is mentioned for historical interest only. In his thesis for the American Orthopaedic Association, Key[9] reviewed the experience with manipulation at the Massachusetts General Hospital for chronic slipped capital femoral epiphysis. Up to this time, manipulation was an accepted treatment. He found that there was *no* correction of the deformity, and all of those which were manipulated ended up with stiff hips. He urged his colleagues to abandon this technique. Manipulation of the acute slipped capital femoral epiphysis, on the other hand, has been less dangerous. Fahey[2] demonstrated that manipulation was a reasonable treatment in patients with a definite, acute, traumatic episode and in whom manipulative treatment was carried out *within 3 weeks* of the acute injury. After manipulation, the hips were fixed with three partially threaded pins. One of ten developed avascular necrosis. In a comprehensive review of British experience, Hall[4] showed all forms of treatment for severe chronic slipped epiphyses are accompanied by various complications. However, neck osteotomy or manipulation and Smith-Peterson nailing give the poorest results. Subtrochanteric osteotomy, although often considered inadequate for complete correction, is the least damaging to circulation. In a thorough review, Howorth[5] pointed out that untreated slipped epiphyses rarely develop aseptic necrosis of the head of the femur and that any treatment given by physicians should help to avoid this complication. He advocated a small cross-epiphyseal graft, a pegging through the plate, in minimal slipped epiphyses. The graft produced little injury to the joint and was effective in preventing additional deformity. This was not widely used, primarily because pinning is less difficult and does not require arthrotomy. We have seen many complications from Knowles pinning in situ (i.e., breakage of the pins, difficulty with removal, and fracture at the base of the pins when trying to remove them). For this reason, we prefer to use wood screws.

Operations through the epiphyseal plate itself were very popular 30 years ago, receiving their stimulus from the work of Klein,[10] who reported superior results. However, since that time, Joplin[8] reported the method to be less successful. Wedge osteotomies of the femoral neck were used by Wilson, Badgley, and others.[1,18,19] The cases without circulatory disturbance gave excellent results, but approximately one third of the patients developed avascular necrosis with very poor results, and this method has been largely abandoned, although the ideal correction would be obtained with an osteotomy placed through the callus at the level of the slip itself. The blood supply to femoral head is extremely vulnerable in this area and makes this procedure prohibitive. More distally along the neck, the incidence of avascular necrosis is not as great. Kramer, Craig, and Noel,[11] Hungrea,[6] and, more recently, Gage[3] have advocated this method, and the short-term results have been encouraging with respect to minimizing the incidence of avascular necrosis. Nevertheless, this complication has occurred in approximately 10% to 20% of the cases.

Another major limitation is the extent of correction obtainable without placing undue stress on the neck. At present, the maximum correction is about 50 degrees and probably is not applicable to completely slipped epiphyses. In addition there is a mechanical disadvantage to be described later. The advantage of the low neck osteotomy is the more direct visualization of the correction itself, but, obviously, since the hip joint is open and the head fragment quite mobile, it is very susceptible to vascular injury, and there are problems with internal fixation.

Osteotomies at or below the lesser trochanter have been carried out for many years, but they have not been popular because it appears conceptually and technically difficult to restore normal anatomic relationships, particularly since the femoral head is not visualized directly. Since this operation is distal to the blood supply, it is the least likely to endanger femoral head circulation. Since 1951 we have used a calibrated, biplane osteotomy through the lesser trochanter, which is safe and effective once the technique is mastered.[16,17] If the anatomic correction is proper, results are excellent.

The major unsolved problem in the management of the slipped capital femoral epiphysis seems to be significant and severe narrowing of the cartilage space.[14] This condition seems more related to the degree of slip, race, and sex, than to treatment modes. Black females with severe slips are the most vulnerable.

MECHANICS OF CORRECTION

Obviously, if one could exactly reverse the deformity with traction to regain length and internal rotation to return the posteriorly tilted varus head into anatomic position, this would be ideal. In a few cases with acute slips, this has been possible only with traction, abduction, and internal rotation. For this reason, we treat all early slips by this method. If they do not correct within 2 weeks, the condition is considered chronic. In a chronic case, some callus or fibrous union has occurred between the neck (epiphyseal) and the neck fragments (metaphyseal). In the cases described by Klein, Joplin, and Reidy,[10] they were able to pry the head back over the epiphyseal plate with astonishing success. In 1952 Dr. Joseph Barr, Sr. demonstrated to one of us how a slipped femoral head could be impaled with a fixation pin while the neck was separated from the base of the epiphysis and internally rotated to restore the epiphyseal arrangement. This operation required an extensive anterior intracapsular dissection, which is difficult in obese patients, and required the utmost caution to avoid injury to the posterior retinaculum. Even without direct damage to the remaining blood supply from manipulation, there is also concern for stretching the posterior capsule to reduce the blood flow present. In addition to these problems, the damage that the surgical procedure may do to the cartilage space is another explanation for failure.[14]

All other neck operations shorten the neck, and if they do not disturb the retinacular blood supply, they do produce some undesirable shortening of the trochanteric musculature, since the trochanter is close to the iliac crest. Shortening of the neck with elevation of the trochanter not only weakens the abductors, but reduces abduction.[12]

On the other hand, if a proper wedge of bone can be removed distal to the greater trochanter and the neck rotated into a valgus position, thus bringing the stuck femoral head into a more valgus and anterior position (reversing the posterior tilt), the distance between the roof of the acetabulum and the trochanter may be restored to normal. However, if the wedge is too large or if the correction of posterior tilt is greater than 45 degrees, this lengthening effect will not occur. Like all other procedures that attempt to restore the valgus position of the head, there is additional pressure on the joint itself. This additional pressure may be responsible for additional narrowing of the cartilage space in some severe cases.

Since the head of the femur remains in the acetabulum and the distal femur goes into marked external rotation, with the trochanter riding high and posterior to the acetabulum, it is possible to carry out a single plane osteotomy at the level of the lesser trochanter, rotating the distal fragment internally. However, this does not restore length to the neck and does not correct the greater trochanter out of its severe posterior position. It is safe from the point of view of circulation of the femoral head, but it weakens the abductors rather severely. This method has been used extensively by Jacobs[7] and his colleagues. We think there is reason to give the greater trochanter better mechanical advantage, and since 1951, we have used the *biplane* method. By a variation in the size of the wedge removed, more or less restoration of the femoral neck length can be ob-

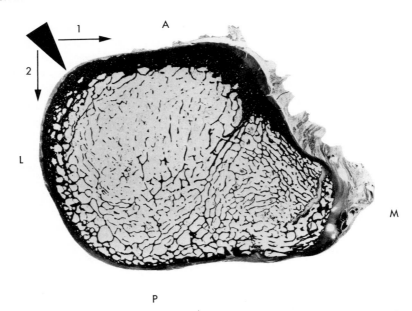

Fig. 6-13. Cross section of femur at level of the lesser trochanter. *A,* anterior; *L,* lateral; *P,* posterior; and *M,* medial. Orientation mark (large arrow) is the demarcation for anterior *(1)* and lateral *(2)* wedge placements.

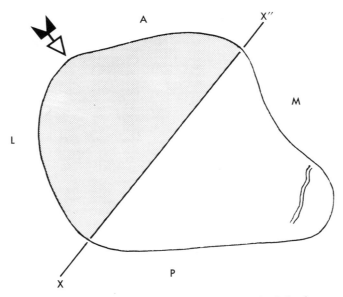

Fig. 6-14. Schematic of transverse section of femur at level of the lesser trochanter. *A,* anterior; *L,* lateral; *P,* posterior; *M,* medial. The stippled area represents the antero-lateral segment of bone to be removed. Approximately 40% to 50% of the bone area is removed.

tained and more or less pressure on the joint cartilage can be applied.

TECHNIQUE OF BIPLANE OSTEOTOMY

The method for this procedure has been thoroughly explained in the past and will be repeated here only briefly, with some minor modifications.[16,17] Recently a fracture table has been used in particularly obese individuals to aid in holding and positioning the limb. Roentgenograms in the AP and lateral positions can be made as in a hip nailing procedure. A skin incision is made laterally along the posterior edge of the femoral shaft and the anterolateral shaft of the femur exposed at the level of the lesser trochanter. At this level, the femur is somewhat rectangular (Fig. 6-13). By checking the knee joint, the anterior surface of the shaft of the femur and the lateral surface of the shaft of the femur can be defined and the confluence of the anterior shaft and the lateral shaft marked (Fig. 6-13). Transverse marks are scribed along the anterior and lateral surfaces where the final osteotomy cut is to be made. The wedge to be cut out can be marked on the anterior and lateral surfaces and the axis point of the wedge also can be defined along the transverse mark (Figs. 6-14 to 6-16). Individuals not wishing to use degrees for calculations can use millimeter measurements. Simply measure 1.5 mm from the transverse mark proximally along the orientation mark (line X-T, Fig. 6-15) and make an oblique line across the anterior shaft (line X''-X, Fig. 6-15). This line will represent the anterosuperior edge of the wedge of bone to be removed. On the lateral surface of the shaft, measure 1.3 mm along the transverse mark (line TX', Fig. 6-16). Then scribe a line from this point (X' to point X, Fig. 6-16). The stippled portion of Figs. 6-15 and 6-16 represent the average amount of bone to be removed. Note that it represents almost the full surface of the anterior shaft and between one half and two thirds of the lateral surface of the shaft (along the transverse line). It should not measure less.

With a bone saw or very sharp osteotome, cut from X to X' along the lateral surface and at the same time follow the scribed line along the anterior surface, X to X'' (Fig. 6-15). The osteotome or saw should follow both of these oblique cuts at the same time, meeting the transverse plane of the femur as seen in Fig. 6-14 (X'-X''), then cutting along the transverse line to remove the wedge. After this oblique wedge of bone has been removed, a fixation pin is placed in the head

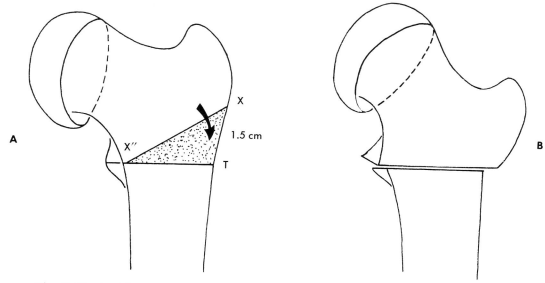

Fig. 6-15. A, After the transverse line has been scribed on the anterior and lateral surface of the bone at the level of the lesser trochanter, the junction of the lateral and the anterior surface is identified and also marked as an orientation mark *(X-T)*. The usual size of wedge to be removed is indicated 1½ cm along the anterolateral orientation mark. **B,** Postoperative position as seen in AP x-ray film.

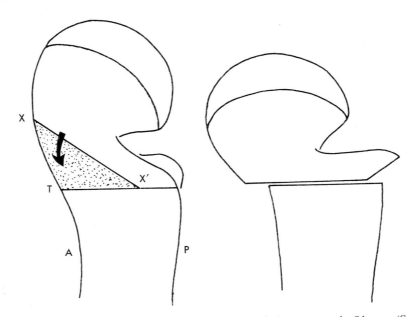

Fig. 6-16. The lateral aspect of osteotomy before and after removal of bone. (See text.)

fragment so that it is possible to control the osteotomy during the application of a side plate. This pin goes roughly parallel to the oblique surface of the osteotomy but is directed toward the lesser trochanter. Now the transverse cut is completed, splitting the lesser trochnter. The wedge of bone removed should be large enough for the upper oblique surface to fit squarely on the lower transverse surface of the distal femur, comprising about 50% of the surface area of the transverse cross section (Fig. 6-14). Since no dissection has occurred posteriorly, the posterior soft tissues act as a hinge. It may be necessary to cut a few of the psoas fibers to allow the hinge enough stretch so that the transverse surface of the lower fragment can fit on the oblique surface of the upper fragment. This is attempted by traction, flexion, and abduction. This can be done with the aid of the fracture table. After closure, the anterior surface of the distal fragment should be touching the anterior surface of the proximal fragment. A compression block is used to hold the fragments in place and guide the drilling of a second holding pin through the distal cortex of the femur about 1 inch from the osteotomy site.[16,17] With the anterior surfaces of the osteotomy cuts aligned, the compression block pulls the two pins together, holding the osteotomy firmly. This difficult part of the procedure can be aided consider

ably with the addition of the fracture table foot support. The completed osteotomy should look like the examples in Figs. 6-15 and 6-16 or Figs. 6-17 and 6-18. Postoperatively, if the plate is holding in tension and there is no movement present at the fracture site, the patient can be placed in bed with pillow support for a few days. Instability of the osteotomy should be determined before closure, and roentgenograms should be made to check the placement of the screws and side plate.

Results

Long-term experience has now been obtained in over 70 hips where a biplane intertrochanteric osteotomy was performed. Using our classification described previously,[16] we had excellent or good results in 87% of the cases, fair results in 8%, and poor results in 5%. The most significant complication, which may not be a complication of the operation itself, is cartilage space narrowing. Cartilage space narrowing of some degree will be visible in one half of the patients with severe slipped epiphysis. In the vast majority, this complication is temporary. We found intermittent rest when the hip was painful and the use of crutches at other times gave the best results. Traction, manipulation, and physical therapy seemed to be of no avail. The incidence of this

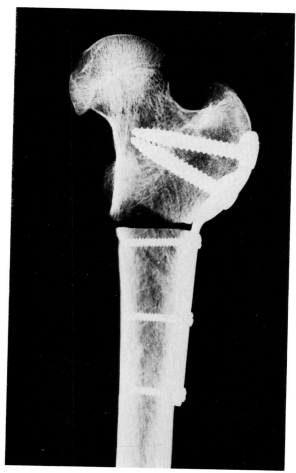

Fig. 6-17. Reduced specimen shows the transverse cut and opening wedge posteromedially. In the clinical situation the plate would be coapted against the proximal fragment under compression. Notice the erect femoral head and tension side plate pulling the trochanter distally, thus giving normal mechanical strength to the abductors and allowing for complete abduction.

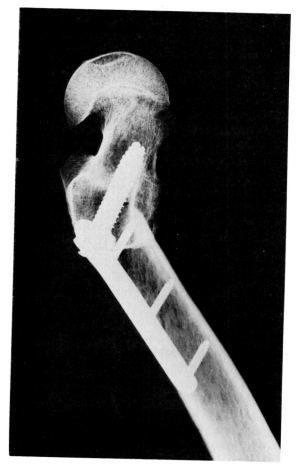

Fig. 6-18. In the lateral plane, tilting the neck anteriorly coapts the full surface of the head of the femur against the acetabulum for weight bearing. Since the head is no longer posteriorly tilted with respect to the shaft, full flexion can be obtained.

problem is higher in blacks and especially in black females.

None of the patients had aseptic necrosis of the head of the femur, and none of them required major reconstructive procedures, such as fusion or joint replacement.

SUMMARY

Some unique anatomic and mechanical aspects of slipped capital femoral epiphysis have been described, along with the rationale for biplane osteotomy correction through the lesser trochanter. Based on long-term experience, we believe bi-

plane osteotomy is the safest form of treatment for the chronic, severe slip because it does not cause avascular necrosis of the head of the femur, does not enter the hip joint, and retains the mechanical advantage of hip abductors.

REFERENCES

1. Badgley, C. E., Isaacson, A. S., Wolgamot, J. C., and Miller, J. N.: Operative therapy for slipped upper femoral epiphysis, J. Bone Joint Surg. **30-A:**19, 1948.
2. Fahey, J. J., and O'Brien, E. T.: Acute slipped capital femoral epiphysis: review of the literature and report of ten cases, J. Bone Joint Surg. **39-B:**659, 1957.
3. Gage, J. R., Sundbert, A. B., Nolan. D. R., Sletten,

R. G., and Winter, R. B.: Complications after cuneiform osteotomy for slipped capital femoral epiphysis, J. Bone Joint Surg. **60-A:**157, 1978.

4. Hall, J. E.: The results of treatment of slipped capital femoral epiphysis, J. Bone Joint Surg. **39-B:**659, 1957.
5. Howorth, M. B.: Slipping of the capital femoral epiphysis, Clin. Orthop. **48:**11, 1966.
6. Hungrea, J.: Pavilhav fernandiho simonsen, Sao Paulo, Brazil, personal communication, 1968.
7. Jacobs, J.: Personal communication, 1962.
8. Joplin, R. J.: Slipped capital femoral epiphysis. The still unsolved adolescent hip lesion, J.A.M.A. **188:**379, 1964.
9. Key, J. A.: Epiphyseal coxa vara or displacement of the capital epiphysis, J. Bone Joint Surg. **8:**53, Jan., 1926.
10. Klein, A., Joplin, R. J., and Reidy, J. A.: Treatment of slipped capital femoral epiphysis, J.A.M.A. **136:**445, 1948.
11. Kramer, W. G., Craig, W. A., and Noel, S.: Compensating osteotomy at the base of the femoral neck for slipped capital femoral epiphysis, J. Bone Joint Surg. **58-A:**796, 1976.
12. Merchant, A. C.: Hip abductor muscle force. An experimental study of the influence of hip position with partic-ular reference to rotation, J. Bone Joint Surg. **47-A:**462, 1965.
13. Ogden, J. A.: Changing patterns of proximal femoral vascularity, J. Bone Joint Surg. **56-A:**941, 1974.
14. Ogden, J. A., Simon, T., and Southwick, W. O.: Cartilage space width and slipped capital femoral epiphysis, Yale J. Biol. Med. **50:**17, 1977.
15. Ogden, J. A., and Southwick, W. O.: Endocrine dysfunction and slipped capital femoral epiphysis, Yale J. Biol. Med. **50:**1, 1977.
16. Southwick, W. O.: Osteotomy through the lesser trochanter for slipped capital femoral epiphysis, J. Bone Joint Surg. **49-A:**807, 1967.
17. Southwick, W. O.: Compression fixation after biplane intertrochanteric osteotomy for slipped capital femoral epiphysis, J. Bone Joint Surg. **55-A:**1218, 1973.
18. Wagner, L. C., and Donovan, M. M.: Wedge osteotomy of the neck of the femur in advanced cases of displaced upper femoral epiphysis. Ten-year study, Am. J. Surg. **78:**281, 1949.
19. Wilson, P. D., Jacobs, B., and Schecter, L.: Slipped capital femoral epiphysis. An end-result study, J. Bone Joint Surg. **47-A:**1128, 1965.

Chapter 7

Orthopaedic aspects of the chronic pain syndrome

DAN M. SPENGLER

JOHN D. LOESER

TERENCE M. MURPHY

Pain related to the musculoskeletal system is the most common symptom causing patients to be directed to an orthopaedist. In the majority of patients, the pain complaints are acute and arise from well-defined traumatic or disease processes. Patients with these acute pain problems generally respond appropriately to traditional medical-surgical treatment, including analgesics, immobilization, and surgery. Patients with chronic pain (6 months or longer), however, pose a more formidable problem for orthopaedists because these patients do not respond to traditional treatment. Furthermore, the subjective symptoms causing patients with chronic pain to seek medical advice are quite similar to the symptoms expressed by patients with acute pain problems. Differentiating the patient with chronic pain from the patient who has acute pain is most important, since management is vastly different.

Although patients with chronic pain complaints represent only a small fraction of the total populace, the cost to society for treating these patients is staggering.[3,6] Bonica[3] has estimated the annual cost in the United States to be between thirty-five and fifty billion dollars. While impressive, these cost estimates do not take into account the cost in terms of human suffering. Although the causes for chronic pain are complex, some of the correctable deficiencies that have been expressed are as follows: (1) failure to apply new knowledge and technology to the study of clinical pain syndromes, (2) improper and inadequate application of current knowledge to the care of chronic pain patients, (3) "tunnel vision," an offshoot of superspecialization, which is reflected in a tendency of the physician to view pain from a very limited perspective, and (4) unwillingness of certain practitioners to devote sufficient time and effort to the management of patients suffering from chronic pain.[3] Other factors that are important in the pathogenesis of chronic pain states include various environmental contingencies (e.g., avoidance of unpleasant tasks, desire for compensation, and pursuit of litigation), which can reinforce the ongoing pain behavior.

The purpose of this chapter is to review the components of chronic pain, to elucidate the clinical characteristics of patients who suffer from chronic pain, and to highlight the pitfalls that confront the physician caring for patients with chronic pain problems. An increased awareness of the unique features of patients suffering from chronic pain, coupled with earlier recognition of patients who are developing chronic pain behavior, will result in an improved assessment and management of these patients.

The majority of chronic pain problems affecting the musculoskeletal system result from operant mechanisms, that is, the pain behavior is strongly influenced by things other than tissue pathology. The two less common causes of chronic pain, persistent noxious stimulation and diseases of the cerebrospinal axis, both respondent mechanisms, will not be dealt with in this chapter.

COMPONENTS OF CHRONIC PAIN

Differentiating acute pain from chronic pain is crucial for proper patient management. The principles of treatment for acute pain problems are ineffective and often counterproductive when applied to patients suffering from chronic pain. The physician must understand that continuing nociception or tissue damage need not be present for pain behaviors to be maintained. Severe pain behaviors can and do occur without any associated tissue irritation or damage.[5] In most patients who suffer from chronic pain, the initial focus for pain (e.g., backache, headache, knee pain) is associated with a relatively minor incident involving nociception (e.g., twisting, lifting, bending). Although the nociceptive focus should resolve rapidly, pain behavior may continue unabated despite treatment that is nearly uniformly effective in other patients. In the case of acute pain such as that produced by striking a finger with a hammer, the resultant pain behavior closely parallels the stimulus (i.e., pain behavior corresponds with nociception) (Fig. 7-1). In the patient with chronic pain, however, thorough multisystem examinations and studies often fail to identify any clear-cut source for the pain behavior. In such instances, nociception does not parallel pain behavior (Fig. 7-1). Clearly, other factors are involved. These factors can be further clarified by examining the components of chronic pain.

The components of chronic pain include nociception, pain sensation, suffering, and pain behavior.[7] Only a very brief outline of the neurophysiology of pain is included in this chapter. The reader is referred to articles by Bonica[3] and Clawson, Bonica, and Fordyce[4] for a more complete discussion of this subject.

Nociceptors are terminals of A delta and C afferent fibers, which, when stimulated, produce discharges that convey information to the central nervous system on the presence of a high-intensity stimulus. Nociceptors can be activated by strong mechanical stimulation, extreme heat (>50° C), or extreme cold (<15° C). The sensation of pain is experienced when nociception is transmitted to the central nervous system. This process results in a sensation labeled as "pain." Clinical pain problems cannot be modeled by this pain sensation alone. Pain sensation activates fibers leading to higher cortical centers, which generate negatively toned affective responses that we label or interpret as "suffering." It is crucial to

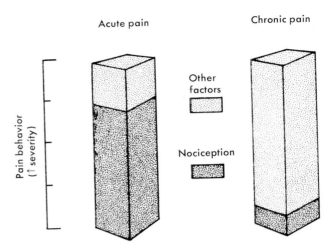

Fig. 7-1. Schematic diagram underscoring the relative contribution of nociception to acute pain and chronic pain.

recognize that suffering can be due to factors other than pain, such as depression, fear, or isolation. "Suffering" in turn, generates pain behaviors (e.g., groaning, writhing, limping). These pain behaviors are the phenomena observed by clinicians when they deal with patients. To repeat, then, this conceptual sequence is *nociception—sensation of pain—suffering—pain behavior.* As individuals progress through this conceptual sequence from nociception through pain behavior, there is increasing opportunity for their behavior to be influenced by factors other than nociception. For example, a patient's prior experience with pain, emotional/affective problems, contingent environmental reinforcements (e.g., sympathy), and the prospect of compensation and litigation can all influence pain behavior. Thus, when we evaluate patients with chronic pain behavior, we must ask which factors or combinations of factors are maintaining the overall pain behavior. Again, it is essential to remember that pain behaviors can occur and continue to occur in the absence of tissue damage (nociception).

CLINICAL CHARACTERISTICS

The clinical characteristics we have identified in patients suffering from chronic pain and our recommendations for dealing with such patients are based on data generated from both the University of Washington Spine Clinic and Pain Clinic. A summary of these characteristics follows:

1. Symptoms lasting longer than 6 months
2. Few, if any, objective findings
3. Medication abuse
4. Difficulty sleeping
5. Depression
6. Manipulative behavior
7. Somatic preoccupations

These patients represent a skewed distribution of recalcitrant patients who have not been improved by numerous treatment attempts by many health care providers. Nevertheless, these patients entered the health care system for an acute pain problem that was unresolved. Awareness of the clinical characteristics of patients with established pain problems should result in the earlier recognition of such patients. Earlier recognition of the patient prone to develop chronic pain will lead to more appropriate management at an earlier point in time and is likely to prevent the entrenched, unsalvageable chronic pain state. The cost involved in the multidisciplinary evaluation and treatment approach outlined here is justified if the following objectives are met in the majority of patients managed: (1) the frequency of these patients' visits to health care providers is decreased, (2) the quantity of medication is reduced, (3) the need for additional surgical procedures is decreased or eliminated, and (4) normal behavior patterns are re-established.

Chronic pain problems vary significantly in history, anatomic location, duration, and frequency. Nevertheless, many patients with clinical pain complaints of 6 months or longer exhibit characteristics that differentiate them from other patients. In general, pain behaviors persist in these patients despite traditional medical and surgical treatment that is usually successful in other patients. The Minnesota Multiphasic Personality Inventory (MMPI) generally reveals a profile characterized by an increase in the t score on scales 1, 2, and 3 (neurotic triad). Despite the paucity of physical findings to support ongoing nociception, these patients militantly deny any possibility that psychosocial factors are important in their overall pain behavior. Such characteristics virtually eliminate these patients from treatment through traditional psychotherapeutic intervention methods.

In general, patients with chronic pain are minimally productive[2] and devote a considerable amount of their time to "doctor shopping." During visits to doctors, chronic pain patients employ various games to achieve their goals (e.g., "I'll bet you can't," "Ain't it awful").[1] Such assaults on the health care delivery system increase the likelihood for inappropriate treatment as complaints persist and time passes. In our experience, the vast majority of patients suffering from chronic musculoskeletal pain abuse medication and are subjected to surgical procedures that do not result in diminishing their pain behavior.[2,10] In fact, many patients complain of increased pain following uneventful technical procedures that are often successful in other patients. Because of the chronicity of the problem and lack of improvement with traditional therapy, chronic pain patients develop behavioral changes including depression, hostility, and an aggressiveness typified by their demanding that the physician "do something."

MEDICATION MISUSE

The majority of patients seeking evaluation of chronic musculoskeletal-related pain complaints abuse medications. Recognition of medication misuse can be quite difficult. Patient histories are often inaccurate, and medications are typically obtained from several physicians. Certain medication abuse problems can be suspected when patients appear inordinately depressed, have slurring of speech, complain that a high percentage of their time is spent lying or sitting, or are too conversant with the names of medication (e.g., the patient requests a specific narcotic for use in pain management). Recognition of excessive medication usage is essential and should be a high priority item for thorough evaluation when chronic pain patients are assessed. Black[2] reported marked improvement in pain behavior in chronic pain patients when they were simply taken off pain-contingent medication and time-contingent medication management was substituted. Detoxification of these patients may on occasion eliminate the necessity for additional evaluations or treatments.

The first step for patients who are taking excessive medications is to obtain an in-hospital drug profile. This profile is obtained by allowing the patient to have any medication requested during the first 24 hours of hospitalization. After this initial profile is taken, the medications that were requested are divided into three groups: narcotics, barbiturates, and others. Each category is accurately converted to an equivalent dosage of methadone, phenobarbital, or other appropriate

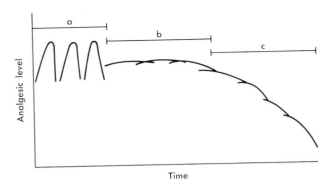

Fig. 7-2. Concept of detoxification medication adjustment. Initially, a drug profile is obtained *(a)*. This process is followed by control with long-acting–time-contingent medications *(b)* and finally withdrawal to a minimum level of analgesic *(c)*. (Modified from Black, R. G.: Surg. Clin. North Am. **55:**1006, 1975.)

long-acting agents to determine the 24-hour requirement of long-acting medications. These medications are then administered in four divided doses in a masking vehicle of constant volume on an exact time-contingency basis (Fig. 7-2). This overall combination approach has been labeled "pain cocktail." The reader is referred to Black's[2] classic article on the chronic pain syndrome for a more detailed discussion of medication adjustment.

One word of caution must be given. Management of these patients is not simple and should be supervised by a physician who is thoroughly familiar with the pharmacology of all medications involved. Monitoring of vital signs is essential, since respiratory arrests may occur when the patient is switched from short-acting medications to longer-acting drugs.

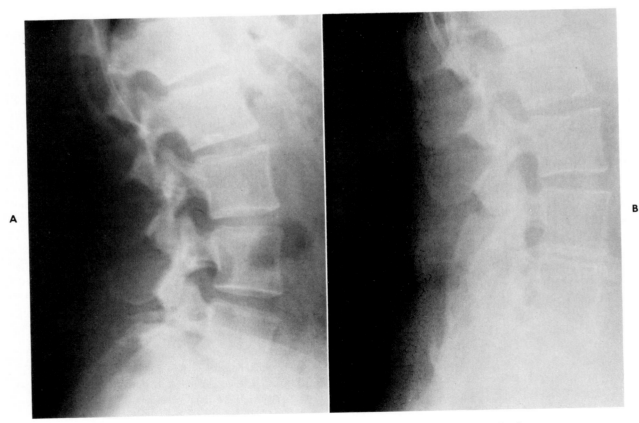

Fig. 7-3. A, Lateral roentgenograms of a patient on initial examination. **B,** Same patient 8 years later after six unsuccessful lumbar spine procedures. Although with the benefit of hindsight, the original procedure was not indicated, an additional seventh procedure may be necessary to decompress a lumbar spinal stenosis caused by the posterior fusion mass.

ASSESSMENT

A major objective during assessment of patients with chronic pain complaints is to determine the role of nociception in the overall pain behavior. In addition to a thorough organic assessment, psychologic testing and a behavioral analysis are performed to determine the contribution of anxiety, depression, and other potential reinforcers of pain behavior. Although an accurate diagnosis is desirable, this ideal cannot always be achieved when patients with chronic pain complaints are evaluated.

During the initial outpatient evaluation, it is useful to have previous medical records available for review. Since the history obtained from the patient is often inaccurate, the past records serve as a cross-check. In most cases, physicians who have treated the patient previously are contacted.

The physical examination of the chronic pain patient must focus on objective findings.[9] Portions of the examination that rely on the response of the patient are generally not reliable, since patient cooperation is often inconsistent. Limited motion of the spine, limping, straight-leg raising, and even "weakness" are all subjective signs that depend on patient cooperation. Psychologic testing and a personal interview by a clinical psychologist or pscyhiatrist are always performed early in the evaluation of chronic pain patients.

After reviewing the past records and interviewing and examining the patient, the clinician can usually outline a reasonable management plan. Since drug detoxification is necessary in most instances, a scheduled hospital admission is arranged. As detoxification is being accomplished, additional diagnostic tests are completed. In the case of chronic low back pain, these tests may include a bone scan, EMG, cystometrogram, and a water-soluble myelogram. Special radiologic studies including tomograms, flexion-extension views, CAT scan, and/or ultrasound are also obtained as indicated.

Diagnostic blocks, performed by a skilled anesthesiologist, are most helpful in the assessment of patients with chronic pain. The graduated spinal block is especially useful in the evaluaton of a patient with chronic back pain and a history of previous surgery. If complete pain relief is obtained following the injection of normal saline in the subarachnoid space, the study is discontinued. This "placebo response" does not rule out the presence of nociception, however, since approx-imately 30% of patients respond in this fashion. Persistence of severe back pain after a complete motor and sensory block is achieved indicates a "central pain" process and implies that surgical intervention is unlikely to benefit the patient.

After completing a thorough multidisciplinary assessment, the key team members meet and outline an appropriate treatment approach. Modalities used can include transcutaneous nerve stimulators, trigger point injections with lidocaine (Xylocaine only), antidepressants, therapeutic nerve blocks, biofeedback, and operant conditioning. Additional surgical intervention is rarely recommended. The 12-month follow-up results of the preceding modalities applied to a group of 65 patients suffering from chronic low back pain were as follows:

1. Ninety percent no longer abused medication and needed no additional surgery.
2. Ten percent received absolutely no value from the treatment and had no improvement; these patients continued doctor shopping and had additional unsuccessful surgeries.

Although results in all patients met the objectives previously outlined, only 6 patients returned to gainful productivity. Thus, the long-term approach to this problem should be earlier recognition, not additional salvage procedures.

Pitfalls

Several pitfalls are commonly encountered during the assessment and treatment of patients suffering from chronic pain. One common misconception is that pain severity should determine how soon to recommend surgical intervention. Since pain is a behavioral phenomenon and can occur in the absence of nociception (tissue damage), surgical intervention based on pain severity can lead to undesirable outcomes, as exemplified in Fig. 7-3. In our experience, the more severe the pain behaviors (e.g., crying, screaming, being unable to move), the less likely we are to find a surgically correctable problem.

Patients who have had chronic pain complaints are quite manipulative and often enlist flattery to obtain their goals (narcotics, surgery). On occasion the patient will bring gifts and suggest that the physician is a superior doctor, unlike all previous doctors, who were not interested in the patient's problem. After such a session, the patient will inevitably request a prescription for a specific

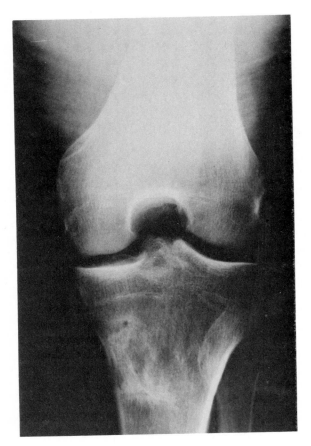

Fig. 7-4. Anteroposterior roentgenogram of the knee of a 28-year-old patient who had three previous knee surgeries that gave no improvement. Because of persistent pain, the patient demanded an amputation. The roentgenogram is normal, as were the results of arthrography and arthroscopy.

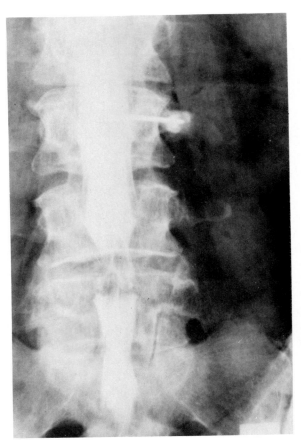

Fig. 7-5. Lumbar myelogram of a 65-year-old woman labeled as a "hysteric" because of a paucity of physical findings. Decompression resulted in a marked decrease in pain behavior.

narcotic or demand that the doctor "do something." An anteroposterior roentgenogram of the knee of such a patient is illustrated in Fig. 7-4. This young man requested an amputation to "cure" his chronic knee pain. Examination revealed a full range of motion with no instability. Results of both arthrography and arthroscopy were within normal limits. In addition, a spinal anesthetic resulting in a complete lower extremity sensory and motor block did not decrease the patient's knee pain. Treatment in an operant conditioning program resulted in a marked decrease in pain behavior and actual return to work.

Short-term pain relief that follows a surgical procedure does not imply that the two events are related. Spangfort[8] reported relief of sciatica in 38% of patients who had negative lumbar disc ex-

plorations. Since placebo responses are not rare, additional surgical procedures should not be recommended solely on the basis of improvement following the first.

On the other hand, patients who have chronic pain complaints and normal physical examinations cannot be assumed to be "hysterical" unless objective evidence exists for such a diagnosis. Patients who suffer from lumbar spinal stenosis are often labeled as having "psychologic problems," since few objective findings are present on a thorough physical examination (Fig. 7-5). Obtaining complete evaluations with electromyography, personality testing, and diagnostic lumbar myelography will further clarify the diagnosis in these patients.

Finally, all attempts should be made to de-

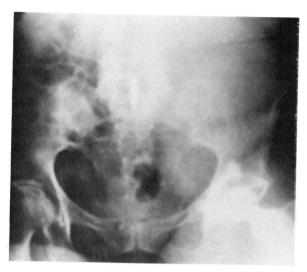

Fig. 7-6. Pelvic roentgenogram of a 62-year-old woman who underwent a decompressive laminectomy and a total hip replacement arthroplasty over a 4-month period, neither of which gave any improvement. Note the large, soft tissue mass in the lower abdominal quadrant on the total hip side. This was a large, recurrent uterine tumor, which likely could have been identified prior to either of the two unsuccessful surgeries.

crease errors in problem solving, such as those illustrated in Fig. 7-6. This woman complained of low back, buttock, and right thigh pain. She underwent a decompression for equivocal lumbar spinal stenosis, which did not alter her pain behavior. Four months later, a total hip replacement arthroplasty was performed with no relief of pain. She was then referred to us for "pain management." A mass the size of a watermelon was noted in the right lower quadrant of the abdomen. After further delineation with ultrasound, surgical exploration demonstrated the mass to be invading the lumbosacral plexus. The mass represented a recurrent uterine tumor. Ob-

taining a complete medical history and performing a pelvic examination prior to her initial decompression would likely have eliminated the necessity for two major surgical procedures. Although earlier recognition of this mass would probably not have altered the prognosis, prompt palliative therapy would have decreased her pain and improved the quality of her life.

SUMMARY

In this chapter we have covered only some of the most important facets of chronic pain. We hope, however, that the general overview presented will stimulate interest in chronic pain problems and provide useful and necessary information to orthopaedists.

REFERENCES

1. Berne, E.: Games people play: the psychology of human relationships, New York, 1964, Grove Press, Inc.
2. Black, R. G.: The chronic pain syndrome, Surg. Clin. North Am. **55:**999, 1975.
3. Bonica, J., editor: Symposium on pain (Parts I and II), Arch. Surg. **112:**749, 783, 861, 1977.
4. Clawson, D. K., Bonica, J. J., and Fordyce, W. E.: Management of chronic orthopaedic pain problems. In The American Academy of Orthopaedic Surgeons: Instructional course lectures, vol. 21, St. Louis, 1972, The C. V. Mosby Co., pp. 8-22.
5. Fordyce, W., Fowler, R., Lehmann, J., and de Lateur, B.: Some implications of learning in problems of chronic pain, J. Chronic Dis. **21:**179, 1968.
6. Johnson, A.: The problem claim, State of Washington, 1978, Department of Labor and Industries (mimeograph).
7. Loeser, J.: Low back pain, Res. Publ. Assoc. Res. Nerv. Ment. Dis. (In press)
8. Spangfort, E.: The lumbar disc herniation, Acta Orthop. Scand. (Suppl) **142:**1, 1972.
9. Spengler, D. M., and Freeman, C. A.: Patient selection for lumbar discectomy: an objective approach, Spine **4:**129, 1979.
10. Spengler, D. M., Freeman, C. A., Westbrook, R., and Miller, J. W.: Low back pain following multiple lumbar spine procedures: failure of initial selection? Spine. (In press)

Chapter 8

Tenosynovial infections in the hand—diagnosis and management

Part I

Acute pyogenic tenosynovitis of the hand

ROBERT J. NEVIASER
STEPHEN F. GUNTHER

Acute tenosynovial infections of the hand are seen with only a moderate degree of frequency. The widespread use of antibiotics for any wound or systemic infection has contributed to the reduction of serious sequelae of bacterial seeding of wounds or the bloodstream. Pyogenic flexor tenosynovitis is one of those unpleasant sequelae, the incidence of which is significantly lower than it was in the preantibiotic era.

Despite the reduced frequency of occurrence, these infections are still present. It is unlikely that flexor tendon sheath infections will be permanently eradicated because of the anatomic nature of these structures.

ANATOMIC CONSIDERATIONS

Doyle and Blythe[3] elucidated the anatomic configuration of the tendon sheath and pulleys in a beautifully detailed study. They noted that the sheaths are double-walled (consisting of a visceral layer or epitenon closely adherent to the tendon and a parietal layer), tubular structures that are hollow. More importantly, the two layers join at the proximal and distal ends, forming a closed or contained system. In the fingers the sheaths begin in the palm at the level of the distal palmar crease or the neck of the metacarpal. They end just proximal to the distal interphalangeal joint.

In the small finger there is usually continuity with the ulnar bursa, which extends into the wrist to a point just proximal to the transverse carpal ligament. In the thumb the sheath communicates with the radial bursa, which extends in a fashion similar to the ulnar bursa, to end just proximal to the carpal tunnel (Fig. 8-1).

Because of their importance as landmarks, the annular pulleys should be noted. There are four of these bands, labeled A1 through A4 by Doyle. A1 is located over the metacarpophalangeal joint, beginning 5 mm proximal to the joint itself. A2 is located over the proximal half of the proximal phalanx. A3 is located at the proximal interphalangeal joint, while A4 is located over the middle third of the middle phalanx (Fig. 8-2). A2 and A4 are the important pulleys to preserve in order to maximize flexor tendon function.

CLINICAL EXAMINATION

The patient usually has a history of a penetrating wound to the involved digit. Personal experience with nearly 40 cases reveals that more than 60% of these patients have had wounds to their fingers or hands. The digits most often involved are the ring, middle, and index fingers.

The four cardinal signs of Kanavel[4] are usually present. These include exquisite tenderness over the course of the flexor tendon sheath, a semiflexed position of the finger (Fig. 8-3, *A*), a sym-

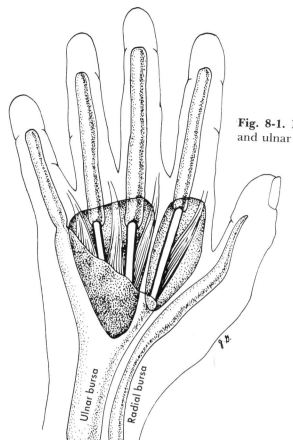

Fig. 8-1. Flexor tendon sheaths and proximal extensions into the radial and ulnar bursae.

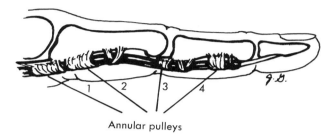

Annular pulleys

Fig. 8-2. Approximate locations of annular pulleys, which are important to flexor tendon function.

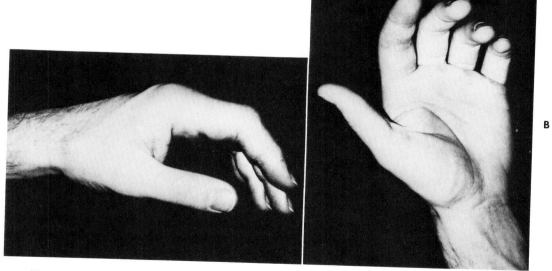

Fig. 8-3. A, Obvious tendon sheath infection with semiflexed position of the finger. **B,** Same patient demonstrating uniform swelling of the index finger from the midpalmar crease to the fingertip. (From Neviaser, R. J.: J. Hand Surg. **3:**462, Sept., 1978.)

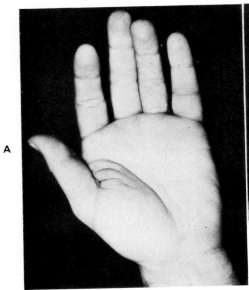

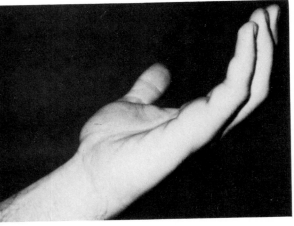

Fig. 8-4. A, Pyogenic flexor tenosynovitis of the small finger demonstrated in a more subtle fashion but not extending into the ulnar bursa. B, The same hand seen from the ulnar side.

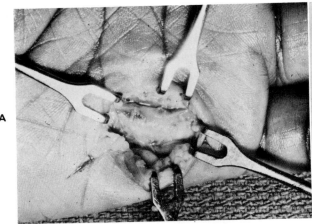

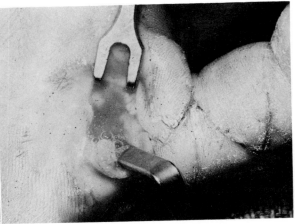

Fig. 8-5. A, Note cloudy serosanguinous fluid in the sheath. This is the usual operative finding. B, Less commonly, overt purulence is encountered.

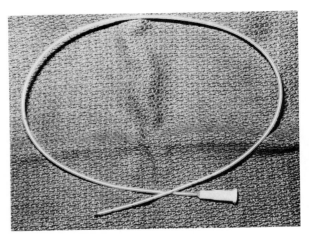

Fig. 8-6. The type of 16-gauge polyethylene catheter used for irrigation of the sheath.

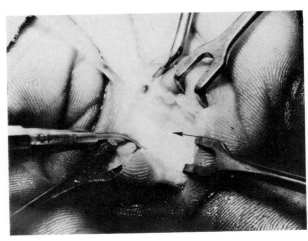

Fig. 8-7. Arrow denotes edge of Al pulley under which catheter is inserted for a distance of 1.5 to 2.0 cm. (From Neviaser, R. J.: J. Hand Surg. 3:463, Sept., 1978.)

metric swelling of the digit (Fig. 8-3, *B*), and marked pain on passive extension of the finger. An additional finding is the inability to flex the finger to touch the palm.

Although some patients may be seen with obvious findings, others may be seen with subtle changes (Fig. 8-4). In the latter group, dependence on eliciting pain with passive extension of the finger has proven the single most reliable sign on which to base a diagnosis. These subtle cases are the ones that are seen relatively early, that is, within the first 72 hours of onset.

TREATMENT

Treatment can be divided into nonoperative and operative forms. The nonoperative approach is applicable only to those cases in which the patient is seen very early in the course of the process. Although a definitive time frame is impossible to establish, a reasonable guideline for classifying a flexor tendon sheath infection as "early" seems to be within 48 hours of onset. I have controlled only four cases by nonoperative means, and all of these were seen within 48 hours after onset.

This form of treatment includes placing the hand at rest in a compressive hand dressing, reinforced by a plaster of paris splint from the fingertips to the proximal forearm, as well as treating the patient with high doses of systemic antibiotics. The choice of antibiotic varies with the treating physician. It is important to recall that

the single most common organism cultured from these patients is *Staphylococcus aureus*. *Pseudomonas aeruginosa* is a distant second. The antibiotic regimen should be selected with this in mind and is ideally administered intravenously while the patient is hospitalized. The finger should be examined at least twice per day, and the process should be nearly resolved within 48 hours.

The operative approach is used for those cases which do not respond to the previously described regimen as well as for those seen later in the course of the disease, usually more than 48 hours after onset. Although several techniques have been described, one method has several advantages over the others. This consists of through-and-through irrigation of the sheath via a closed system using a catheter. The advantages of this method are that it provides a rapid and complete return of function and causes minimal inconvenience to the patient.

Since the first recommended use of catheters in treating infections of the hand,[2] reports of success with their use have been dramatic but not widely appreciated. The technique that will be described has been used successfully in 35 cases.[5] In the operative room, with the patient under general anesthesia and with appropriate preparation including the use of a tourniquet, a zigzag incision is made in the palm over the proximal edge of the tendon sheath. Usually cloudy serosanguineous fluid is seen within the sheath (Fig. 8-5, *A*), although overt purulence may be encoun-

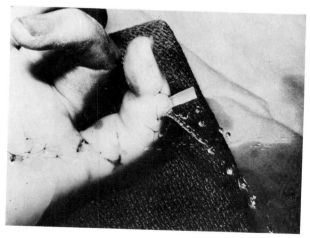

Fig. 8-8. When a wound is irrigated proximally to distally with saline, a free flow should appear from the distal wound. (From Neviaser, R. J.: J. Hand Surg. **3:**463, Sept., 1978.)

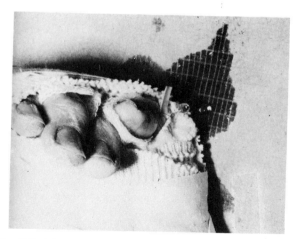

Fig. 8-9. Visualization of the drain in the postoperative dressing allows for the supervision of the manual irrigation. (From Neviaser, R. J.: J. Hand Surg. **3:**463, Sept., 1978.)

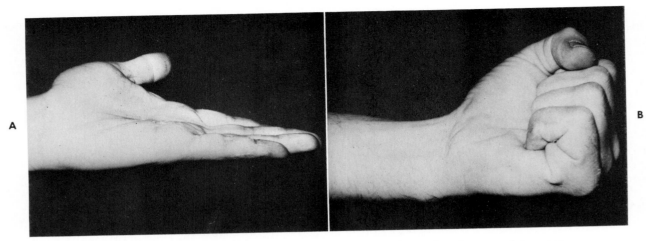

Fig. 8-10. A, One week after drainage and irrigation, the patient has complete extension of the involved small finger. **B,** There is also complete active flexion. (From Neviaser, R. J.: J. Hand Surg. **3:**464, Sept., 1978.)

tered (Fig. 8-5, *B*). Part of the sheath proximal to the Al pulley is excised, and the fluid is cultured. The distal portion of the sheath is exposed through an ulnar midaxial incision in the middle and distal segments of the finger (for the thumb, the radial side should be used). The sheath is excised distal to the A4 pulley. A 16-gauge polyethylene catheter approximately 25 cm long (Fig. 8-6) is inserted proximally to distally under the A1 pulley in the palm for a distance of 1.5 to 2 cm (Fig. 8-7). After insertion of a small rubber drain into the distal wound down to the sheath, the respective wounds are closed. Saline is then flushed from the proximal to the distal end (Fig. 8-8). A compressive dressing with a dorsal plaster splint is applied, and the catheter is brought out of the dressing. Around the fingertip, the dressing is arranged to allow visualization of the rubber drain (Fig. 8-9). The sheath is flushed again before the patient leaves the operating suite.

Postoperatively, the sheath is irrigated with 50 ml of sterile saline every 2 hours for 48 hours. This must be done manually, since a gravity drip does not have a sufficient pressure gradient to irrigate this small space. Systemic antibiotics are also used. After 2 days the digit is inspected. If there are no longer any of the cardinal signs, then the catheter and drain are removed. If one is suspicious that there is persistent infection, the irrigation may continue for 24 to 48 hours more.

When the catheter and drain are removed, the

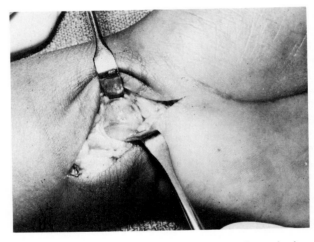

Fig. 8-11. Exposure of the ulnar bursa at the wrist in a case with bursal involvement.

wounds are dressed lightly, and active motion is started. One can expect complete active and passive motion within 1 week of drainage (Fig. 8-10).

Slight modifications are needed for the thumb and small finger. In the thumb the catheter is placed into the radial bursa at the wrist and threaded into the sheath of the flexor pollicis longus as it leaves the carpal canal. In the small finger the ulnar bursa may not be involved, but if it is (Fig. 8-11), then a dual irrigating system can be used. One catheter is placed under the A1 pulley, as already described, to irrigate distally. The sec-

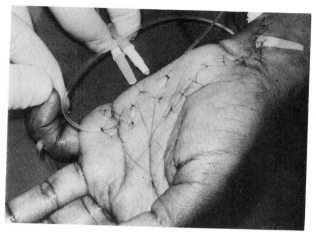

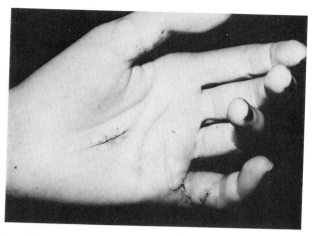

Fig. 8-12. Use of double catheter system for cases with involvement of the bursa as well as the digital sheath. One catheter is directed distally from the palm, while the other is oriented proximally. Small rubber drains provide exit portals for saline in the finger and at the wrist.

Fig. 8-13. A few days following flexor tendolysis, this patient developed a tendon sheath infection. (From Neviaser, R. J.: J. Hand Surg. **3:**464, Sept., 1978.)

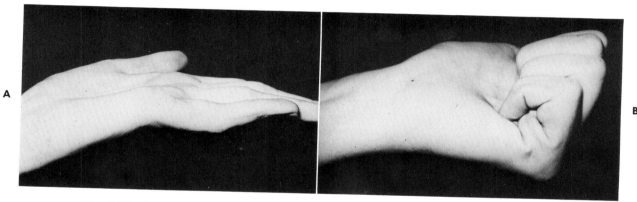

Fig. 8-14. A, Six months postoperatively the patient has a 10-degree flexion contracture at the proximal interphalangeal joint. **B,** Complete flexion is present, however. (From Neviaser, R. J.: J. Hand Surg. **3:**465, Sept., 1978.)

ond is directed proximally in the palm, and a drain is inserted at the wrist for the egress of the retrograde irrigation (Fig. 8-12).

This method has been used to salvage surgical procedures.[5] A young woman, who had undergone flexor tendolysis 6 months after a delayed primary repair of the flexor profundus to the small finger, developed a tendon sheath infection a few days postoperatively after starting exercises (Fig. 8-13). Just prior to tendolysis her total active motion was 190 degrees, while her total passive motion was 245 degrees. She was treated in the described operative manner and showed improved active motion within one week. Six months later her total passive motion was 255 degrees, and her total active motion was 245 degrees (Fig 8-14).

Although two other methods are used currently, each presents a risk for potentially disastrous complications. The use of a single palmar or digital incision for catheter introduction, using this portal to instill saline or antibiotics, does not provide adequate evacuation of necrotic debris and purulence (Fig. 8-15, *A* and *B*). Since the

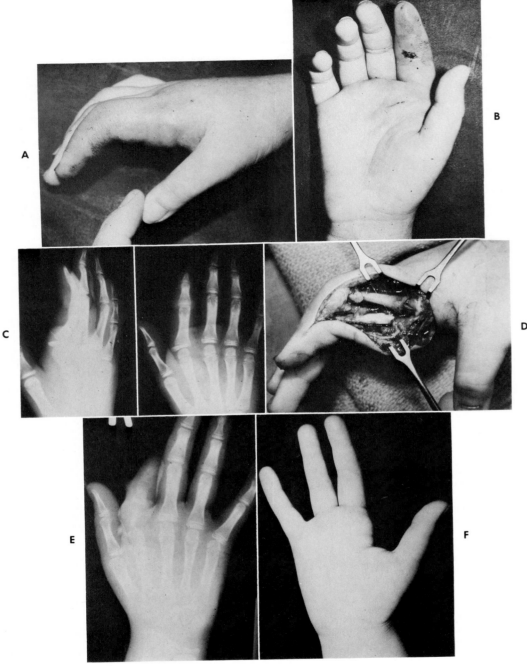

Fig. 8-15. A and **B,** A 10-year-old child with a grossly infected finger following an attempt to drain and irrigate the flexor sheath through a single incision. **C,** Accompanying roentgenogram here showed epiphyseal separation due to infection. **D,** At exploration, the phalanx and tendon were infected and ischemic. **E,** Despite attempts to save the digit, the osteomyelitis continued to progress. **F,** A ray amputation terminated a prolonged and morbid course for the patient, with a useful hand resulting. (From Neviaser, R. J.: J. Hand Surg. **3:**465, Sept., 1978, and Neviaser, R. J., and Adams, J. P.: In Epps, C. H., editor: Complications in orthopaedic surgery, ed. 1, Philadelphia, 1978, J. B. Lippincott Co.)

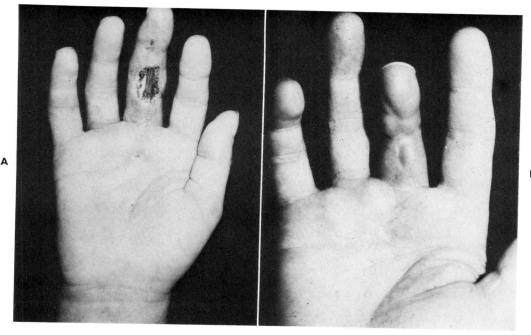

Fig. 8-16. A, Skin flap loss and tendon necrosis resulted from open treatment of this tendon sheath infection. **B,** Shortening the digit by proximal interphalangeal joint fusion salvaged use of the digit, although ablation would have been preferable. (From Neviaser, R. J.: J. Hand Surg. **3:**465, Sept., 1978, and Neviaser, R. J., and Adams, J. P.: In Epps, C. H., editor: Complications of orthopaedic surgery, ed. 1, Philadelphia, 1978, J. B. Lippincott Co.)

tendon already suffers from impaired blood supply due to the increased intrathecal pressure, this approach risks further ischemic damage to the tendon as well as extension into the adjacent phalanges, resulting in an additional osteomyelitis (Fig. 8-15, *C* to *E*). In the presence of this difficult combination, the best option often is amputation (Fig. 8-15, *F*).

The technique of extensive exposure, resection of the sheath, and closure by secondary intention not only prolongs rehabilitation but may cause necrosis of the skin flaps and the flexor tendon (Fig. 8-16, *A*). While ablation is also a reasonable salvage procedure in the face of this complication, sometimes shortening the finger via proximal interphalangeal joint fusion will accomplish closure and leave a moderately useful digit (Fig. 8-16, *B*).

DIFFERENTIAL DIAGNOSIS

The diagnosis of acute tenosynovial infection in the hand is rarely difficult to differentiate from other processes. If one looks for the four cardinal signs, the condition is usually obvious.

On occasion, an acute inflammatory reaction to local calcific deposits may cause some confusion (Fig. 8-17, *A*). The signs of inflammation and other findings associated with infection may be present. There is, however, rarely a history of a penetrating wound, and the roentgenogram provides the correct diagnosis (Fig. 8-17, *B* and *C*).

Acute episodes of gout may be present in the hand, but this is rarely found. The findings are usually not as severe as with an infection but can be such that exploration is undertaken. At surgery the presence of gouty deposits in the absence of cloudy synovial fluid in the sheath should help establish the pathologic nature of the process.

Cellulitis, localized subcutaneous abscesses, furuncles, felons, and paronychia are all readily differentiated from more serious infections. Dactylitis associated with Reiter's syndrome or acute tenosynovitis due to other collagen vascular diseases rarely should be confusing. The history and

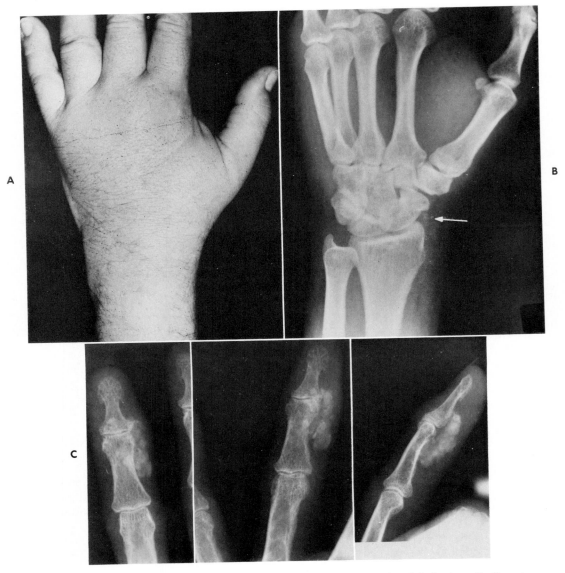

Fig. 8-17. A, A red, swollen, and painful hand, which simulated infection. **B,** Roentgenogram revealed calcific deposits at the wrist (arrow). **C,** Another massive calcific deposit (tumoral calcinosis), which can appear to be a tendon sheath infection.

other evidence of joint involvement should be present. Osteomyelitis will show roentgenographic signs within a week, which is approximately the point at which it may begin to stimulate pyogenic tenosynovitis.

It should never be necessary to attempt to aspirate a tendon sheath in order to establish a diagnosis.

SUMMARY

Acute pyogenic tenosynovial infections of the hand involve virtually only the flexor tendons. The diagnosis should be readily established using clinical findings and the history. If the process is of less than 48-hour duration, nonoperative treatment can be successful, but if this fails or the infection has been present longer, through-and-through irrigation of the sheath as described will provide an excellent result.

REFERENCES

1. Carter, S. J., Burman, S. O., and Mersheimer, W. L.: Treatment of digital tenosynovitis by irrigation with peroxide and oxytetracycline, Ann. Surg. **163**:645, 1966.
2. Dickson-Wright, A.: Tendon sheath infection, Proc. R. Soc. Med. **39**:504, 1943-1944.
3. Doyle, J. R., and Blythe, W.: The finger flexor tendon sheath and pulleys: anatomy and reconstruction. In American Academy of Orthopaedic Surgeons: Symposium on tendon surgery in the hand, St. Louis, 1975, The C. V. Mosby Co., pp. 81-87.
4. Kanavel, A. B.: Infections of the hand, ed. 7, Philadelphia, 1943, Lea & Febiger, pp. 241-242.
5. Neviaser, R. J.: Closed tendon sheath irrigation for pyogenic flexor tenosynovitis, J. Hand Surg. **3**:462, 1978.

Part II

Chronic tenosynovial infections in the hand

STEPHEN F. GUNTHER
ROBERT J. NEVIASER

A discussion of chronic tenosynovial infection is really a discussion of infection by mycobacteria, principally the nontuberculous mycobacteria. These "atypical" organisms have been considered opportunistic pathogens, but the increasingly frequent identification of *Mycobacterium marinum*, *Mycobacterium kansasii*, and *Mycobacterium avium* or *intracellulare* (Battey bacillus) infections attest to their virulence in normal hosts. Table 6 presents the atypical mycobacteria that are at least potentially pathogenic to humans. They cause pulmonary and extrapulmonary diseases similar to tuberculosis. An excellent general review of the nontuberculous mycobacteria and their associated diseases has recently been written by Wolinsky.[13]

We have had experience with 8 cases of atypical mycobacteria infections and 1 case of tuberculous infection in the synovial spaces of the hand and wrist. Some of these have been reported previously.[4,5] Our cases consist of 4 *M. marinum*, 2 *M. kansasii*, and 2 Group III organisms, presumably *M. avium* or *intracellulare*. *M. marinum* infections are much more predominant in the literature and in a recent survey of hand surgeons. Eighty-six hand surgeons have responded to a questionnaire

Table 6. The Runyon classification*†

I. Photochromogens	*M. kansasii*
	M. marinum
	M. simiae
II. Scotochromogens	*M. scrofulaceum*
	M. szulgai
III. Nonchromogens	*M. avium*
	M. intracellulare
	M. ulcerans
	M. xenopi
IV. Rapid growers	*M. fortuitum*
	M. chelonei

*Slightly modified from Gunther, S. F., Elliott, R. C., Brand, R. L., and Adams, J. P.: J. Hand Surg. **2**(2):91, 1977.
†These mycobacteria are considered at least potentially pathogenic to man.[11] *M. avium* complex includes *M. avium* and *M. intracellulare*, which are extremely similar. *M. marinum*, *M. kansasii*, and *M. avium* complex have been reported in hand infections.

sent to members of the American Society for Surgery of the Hand.[3] Thirty-one had treated mycobacterial infections of the hand, and 45 had not. There were 40 cases of atypical mycobacterial infections and 9 cases of tuberculous infections. When we combined these with cases previously reported[1,7-10,12] and our cases that have not been reported, we found the following kinds of infections: 55 *M. marinum*, 11 *M. kansasii*, 9 Group III (presumably these are *M. avium* or *intracellulare*), and 6 undetermined. *M. marinum* infections come from punctures in a marine environment. The vast majority of cases come from the eastern and southern seaboards, warm freshwater lakes, and household tropical fish tanks. The source of infection of the other organisms is moot. *M. kansasii* infections seem to be more common in the central United States. Some of these infections are associated with punctures, and some are not. Both *M. kansasii* and *M. avium* or *intracellulare* cause pulmonary disease and theoretically could spread by a hematogenous route.

CASE REPORTS

Two of our cases are presented in detail and followed with a general discussion of the clinical presentation, differential diagnosis, and management of the problem.

Case 1

In November, 1976, we treated a 61-year-old, white, male dentist with chronic flexor tenosynovitis in the right long finger. The problem began approximately 4 years previously with a thorn puncture-laceration to the fingertip. The tip became acutely inflamed, and the patient was treated with antibiotics. The inflammation subsided somewhat, but more of the finger became involved. The patient was treated inter-mittently with rest and antibiotics on several occasions. An aspiration of the finger at 18 months grew scant colonies of *Staphylococcus epidermidis*. For the next 2½ years, the finger remained swollen, but the patient sought no further medical help.

Examination revealed that the finger was swollen cir-

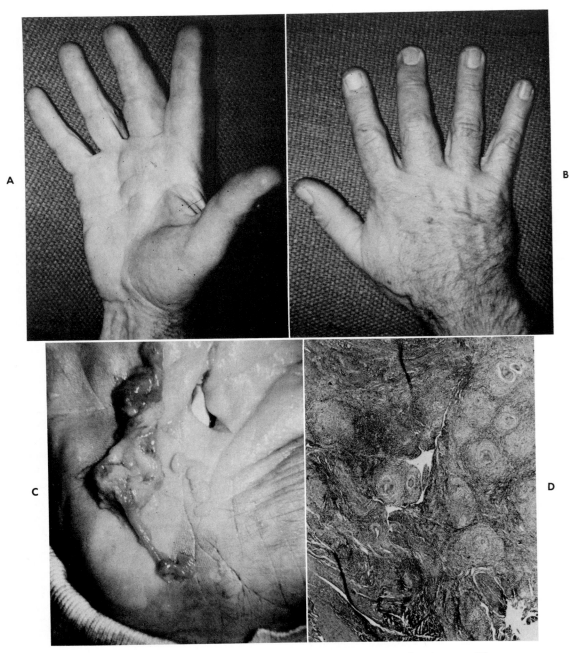

Fig. 8-18. A 61-year-old dentist suffered with a swollen finger for 4 years. Biopsy revealed proliferative synovium and loose bodies. Histology showed an obvious granulomatous synovitis. At follow-up, the patient is completely healed. (See text.)

cumferentially although the flexor tenosynovial space seemed definitely to be the origin of the problem (Fig. 8-18, *A* and *B*). The synovial space in the palm was swollen. Flexion was limited, and there was crepitus within the sheath. The finger was neither red nor warm. There was no obvious wound at the fingertip, no drainage, and no involvement of other fingers or the wrist.

Roentgenograms of the hand were normal except for a suggestion of some periosteal reaction along the volar aspect of the proximal phalanx of the long finger. Fungal skin tests were negative. PPD-S* (*M. tuberculosis*) was positive at 13 mm; PPD-Y (*M. kansasii*) was also positive at 13 mm, and PPD-B (*M. intracellulare*) was negative. Complete blood count (CBC) was negative, and a chest x-ray film showed no abnormalities.

With the idea that this was a *Mycobacterium kansasii* infection that would be quite susceptible to antituberculous medications and considering the patient's busy dental practice, we carried out an excisional biopsy of the palmar portion of the synovial sheath with the patient under local anesthesia in December, 1976. All synovium was removed from the lumbrical origin proximally to the midportion of the A1 tendon sheath pul-

---

*PPD-S is the standard purified protein derivative (Mantoux), intermediate strength, that is used for skin testing. PPD-Y is a specially prepared antigen, which is more specific for *M. kansasii*. PPD-B is more specific for *M. intracellulare*.

ley distally. The sheath was full of yellow fluid, exuberant synovium, and rice bodies (Fig. 8-18, *C*).

Histologic sections confirmed a granulomatous synovitis without caseation (Fig. 8-18, *D*). Fluorochrome examination revealed no acid-fast organisms. Immediately after surgery the patient began triple drug therapy consisting of 300 mg isoniazid, 600 mg rifampin, and 1200 mg ethambutol daily.

The wound healed primarily. At 16 days, *M. marinum* grew on culture. Complete surgical synovectomy was then recommended, but the patient declined because of his professional commitments. By 8 weeks, finger swelling had decreased and motion was good.

In vitro sensitivities showed resistance to isoniazid and sensitivity to rifampin and ethambutol. The patient again declined complete surgical synovectomy, since he felt he was improving without it. He was completely asymptomatic at 13 months. There was no swelling in the finger, and there was no crepitus on motion. There was minimal tendon adherence; he lacked only the final 10 degrees of total active flexion in the finger (Fig. 8-18, *E* and *F*). The drugs were continued for 24 months. The patient is still asymptomatic 30 months after beginning treatment.

Case 2

A 54-year-old white housewife was referred for evaluation in November, 1976. She had been treated with prednisone for 20 years because of her asthma. She

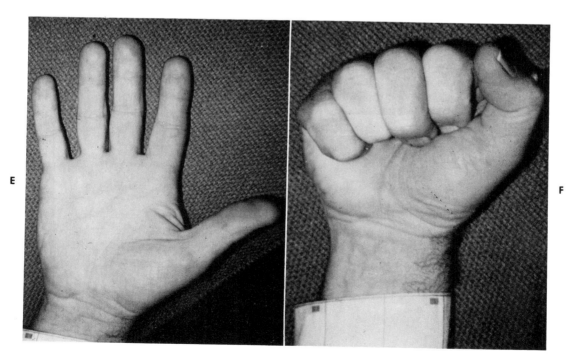

Fig. 8-18, cont'd. For legend see opposite page.

had an open wound in the right palm from a previously diagnosed Group III mycobacterial infection (Fig. 8-19, *A*). The finger was slightly swollen, and the ruptured ends of flexor tendons were visible in the ulcer.

She had sustained blunt trauma to the right long finger 2 years previously while rowing in the Potomac River. She could recall no laceration. Pain and stiffness developed over the next 6 months. Steroids were injected into the flexor tendon sheath on many occasions over the next 18 months. There was temporary relief of swelling and ache each time. Trials of antibiotic were of no help. There were no systemic symptoms at any time. In July, 1976, incision had been made in the palm, and partial tenosynovectomy was performed as a biopsy. The histology revealed necrotizing granulomas consistent with tuberculous infection. Initial smears did not show any acid-fast organisms, but a fluorochrome stain later did. Within a few weeks, treatment was instituted with 300 mg isoniazid, 600 mg rifampin, 1200 mg ethambutol. The wound broke down 6 weeks after surgery and grew *Staphylococcus epidermidis*. The use of isoniazid was discontinued in October, 1976, because of a drug hepatitis.

In November, 1976, surgery was performed by one of us (S. F. G.). The whole tendon sheath and the tendons were removed (Fig. 8-19, *B*). Some of the granulomatous tissue had grown out of the sheath and into the interosseous space between the long and ring fin-

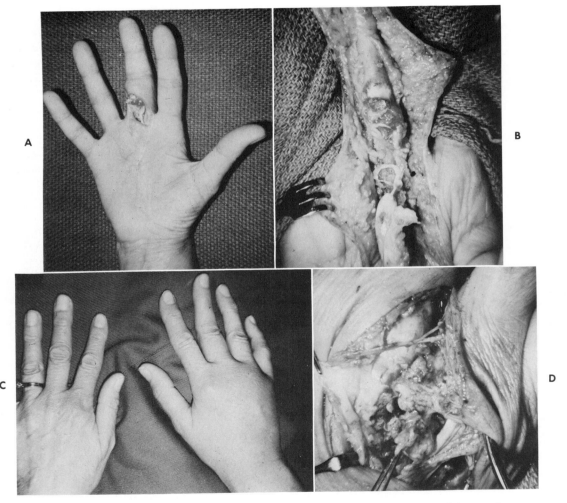

Fig. 8-19. A 54-year-old housewife with ruptured flexor tendons exposed in an ulcer. Synovial debris was removed surgically from the palm and finger, but a dorsal abscess developed in the subaponeurotic space, which required drainage. A cystic abscess was later removed from the web space. The hand appears to be free of disease at 33 months. (See text.)

gers. As much of this as could be reached through the volar incision was excised. Histology again revealed caseating granulomas. No organisms were seen. A non-chromogenic niacin-negative mycobacterium grew in 4 weeks. At 6 weeks, the wounds were well-healed, and the hand looked fine. By 11 weeks, there was significant dorsal swelling (Fig. 8-19, *C*) and pain on passive flexion of the long finger. There was marked intrinsic tightness. A large amount of pus was obtained through a needle, and this was found to contain acid-fast organisms. The oral prednisone dosage had been increased during this postoperative period due to exacerbation of the asthma.

Surgery was again performed in February, 1977. A

dorsal incision was made along the third ray covering proximally to cross the ring and little finger metacarpals. Infected synovium and pus were debrided from the subaponeurotic space under the extensor tendons (Fig. 8-19, *D*). The infected interosseous muscles between the long and ring finger ray were completely excised. There was no apparent osteomyelitis. Smear was positive for organisms, but none grew on culture at this time. Streptomycin was added to the drug program for 3 weeks at which time its use was discontinued because the patient became dizzy. The wound healed primarily except for a delay at the drain site in the web space.

By November, 1977, the wounds were mobile, and

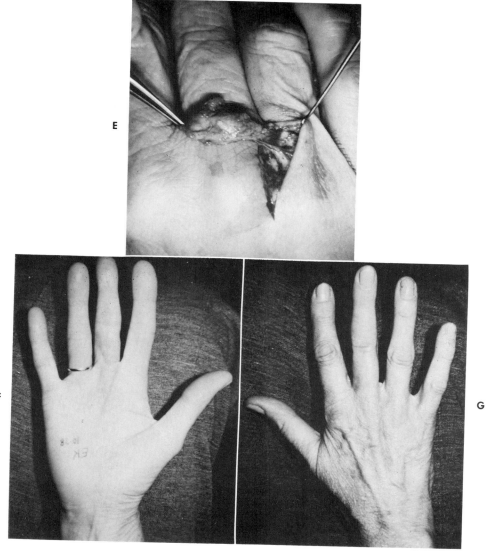

Fig. 8-19, cont'd. For legend see opposite page.

there was no swelling in the hand. There was no sign of persistent infection. There was full mobility of all fingers except for the long finger, which was quite stiff in extension. The patient eventually noticed two small cystic masses, one in the web space between the long and ring fingers and one in the old palmar incision. These were excised in March, 1978, and proved to be encapsulated abscesses (Fig. 8-19, E). Histology again revealed caseating granulomas, but no organisms were seen or grown on culture.

The antituberculous drugs were discontinued after 24 months. Two years and 9 months after diagnosis, the hand appears to be free of disease with the exception of two small firm nodules in the palmar incision. These could be two more cystic abscesses. Otherwise, the volar and dorsal wounds are fine (Fig. 8-19, F and G). During this whole course, the patient had suffered two other infections, which she healed without treatment. One was a mixed infection of a leg wound, and the other was a staphylococcal paronychia.

CLINICAL PRESENTATION

From the survey of hand surgeons, it is obvious that the diagnosis of atypical mycobacterial infection has been made much more frequently in the past 3 or 4 years than previously. In the past, most patients were diagnosed incorrectly and treated inappropriately for at least 6 months in the beginning of their clinical course. This is changing now, and the diagnosis is being made earlier.

Patients are typically middle-aged, and most are healthy, contrary to the belief that atypical mycobacteria prey only upon the immunologically deficient. This is particularly so with *M. marinum*, which will infect anyone. Two of our 8 patients were immunologically depressed, one from chronic steroid treatment for systemic lupus erythematosus, and the other was the patient discussed in Case 2. We feel that *M. marinum* is always introduced by direct inoculation. The organism will not survive at body core temperature and is found only in skin and in the hand. In some cases, the other mycobacteria are inoculated directly through puncture wounds and lacerations, but some appear to spread by a hematogenous route.

Of the cases in the literature, carpal tunnel syndrome with or without involvement of a finger was found in half the cases. This has been the case in only one of our patients. The infection spreads along synovial spaces. One of our patients developed *M. kansasii* infection, which spread along a classic horseshoe pattern involving the little finger, the ulnar and radial bursae in the palm and wrist, and the thumb. The disease is generally indolent, but persistent. Anti-inflammatory agents may give temporary partial remission. Appropriate treatment will cure the problem in most cases. Residual disability after treatment may range from almost nothing to severe, as in the two cases already presented.

Intradermal skin testing with intermediate strength purified protein derivative (PPD) gave no reaction in 4 of our patients. There is cross-reactivity between *M. tuberculosis* and the atypical mycobacteria, and skin tests have been more helpful in most of the published reports. A positive skin test is significant, but a nonreactive test certainly does not mean that a mycobacterial infection is not present. Differential skin testing with antigens supposedly more specific for individual mycobacteria have not been helpful. These different antigens are not even available in most places.

DIFFERENTIAL DIAGNOSIS

Although there may be more, the principal differential diagnoses of the atypical mycobacteria are listed below:

1. Tuberculosis
2. Gout
3. Rheumatic synovitis
4. Fungal infection

M. tuberculosis infections are identified and treated in the same way as the atypical mycobacterial infections. We have seen one 45-year-old man with twice recurrent tuberculous synovitis in the first extensor compartment of the wrist. Undoubtedly, many cases of atypical mycobacterial infection have been diagnosed as tuberculosis in the past.

We have seen one case of gout that resembled the clinical picture of atypical mycobacterial infection. This was in a 64-year-old alcoholic man who experienced a swollen long finger of 1-year duration (Fig. 8-20, A). The gross appearance of his synovium was different from that of the mycobacterial infections (Fig. 8-20, B), and the histopathology was much more typical of gout (Fig. 8-20, C). Antituberculous medication was not started, and the diagnosis of gout was made with confidence 5 days after surgery when he developed acute olecranal bursitis with a crystalline effusion.

We have seen 3 cases of localized flexor teno-

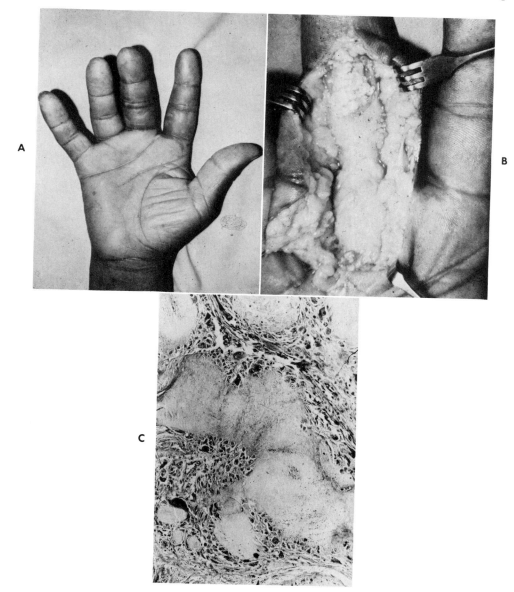

Fig. 8-20. A 64-year-old alcoholic with a chronic gouty tenosynovitis. The gross appearance and histology are different from those of granulomatous infections. (See text.)

synovitis that we consider to be of rheumatic origin. A definite diagnosis has not been made in any of these cases, although a presumptive diagnosis of seronegative rheumatoid arthritis was made in 2 cases. A case in point is a 26-year-old woman who had developed index tenosynovitis of 8-month duration (Fig. 8-21, *A*). She recalled a laceration to the fingertip and a mild paronychial infection at the onset. At surgery, the amount of synovium was less than in the mycobacterial infec-

tions (Fig. 8-21, *B*). There were no rice bodies and no granulomas on biopsy.

Fungal tenosynovitis is extremely rare. To our knowledge only 2 cases have been reported.[2,6] All fungal infections in the hand are rare, and when they occur, they are usually in the form of an abscess or ulceration in the skin, subcutaneous tissue, and sometimes bone. Sporotrichosis, with multiple draining scores along a lymphangitic pattern, is the most common.

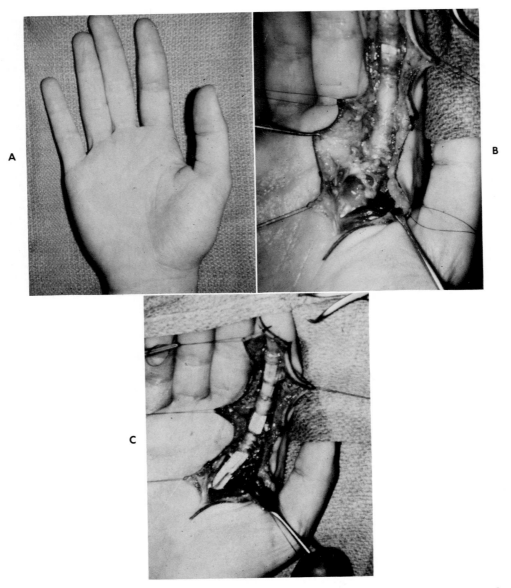

Fig. 8-21. A, A 26-year-old woman with localized index tenosynovitis, probably of rheumatic origin. **B,** The gross appearance and histology of the synovium are different from those of mycobacterial infections. **C,** The flexor sheath pulleys are not involved in the disease.

We have not seen chronic tenosynovitis from foreign material, although this is conceivable, and we have not seen it from other causes.

MAKING THE DIAGNOSIS

Surgical biopsy is imperative in making the diagnosis in cases of chronic tenosynovial infection. If a mycobacterial infection is to be treated, the specific organism must be identified for drug-sensitivity testing. We feel that an unremitting localized synovitis that does not fit a rheumatoid or gouty pattern should be biopsied. This includes inflamed synovium encountered in carpal tunnel release procedures. Histopathologic slides must be reviewed by both the surgeon and the pathologist with a high index of suspicion. A granulomatous synovitis is a key factor, and visualization of the organisms with special stains assures the

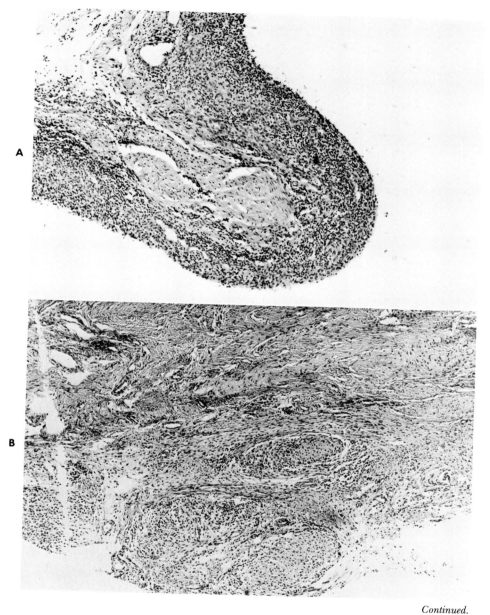

Continued.

Fig. 8-22. Three consecutive synovial biopsies from the long finger of a 34-year-old mechanic. **A,** Although rice bodies were found, the first biopsy shows no evidence of granuloma formation. There is chronic synovitis. **B,** At the second biopsy, 6 months later, one microscopic field showed some poorly differentiated granulomas. These were not appreciated.

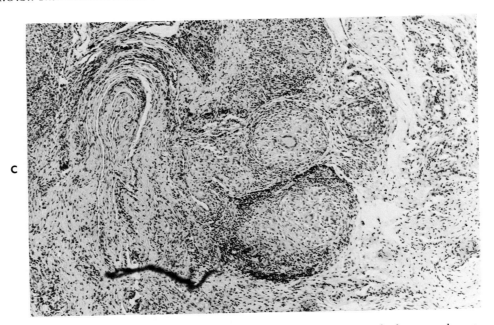

Fig. 8-22, cont'd. C, At the third biopsy, 1 year after the second, the granulomatous nature of the synovitis is obvious. (From Gunther, S. F., Elliott, R., Brand, R., and Adams, J.: J. Hand Surg. **2:**92, Mar., 1977.)

diagnosis. In three of our cases, the significance of unimpressive granuloma formation was not appreciated initially by the pathologist. Such a case is shown in Fig. 8-22. This 31-year-old man underwent excisional biopsy on three different occasions. The first time, there was no granuloma formation seen in a limited specimen (Fig. 8-22, *A*). Months later, there was only one microscopic field showing granuloma formation (Fig. 8-22, *B*), and this was not the typical well-developed granuloma of tuberculosis. It was overlooked. After another year, a third biopsy showed a textbook picture of noncaseating granulomas (Fig. 8-22, *C*).

Special stains must be done for mycobacteria, fungi, and crystals. The mycobacteria are difficult to see even in heavy infection. The modern fluorochrome technique improves yield. Silver stains will show most of the fungi, but not all. Gout does have a characteristic appearance on hematoxylin and eosin stain, but absolute identification depends upon the surgeon having preserved some of the specimen in alcohol for examination under polarized light.

Cultures must be grown for both mycobacteria and fungi in all cases. Although clinicians and pathologists are becoming more aware of atypical mycobacteria, the laboratory still must be advised to incubate the cultures at 31° C as well as the standard 37° C because *M. marinum* will usually grow at the lower temperature only. Many small laboratories are not equipped for this and are particularly not equipped to perform differential cytochemical tests for species identification. If this is the case, the specimen should be sent to a larger laboratory.

Seeing a mycobacterium, fungus, or collection of crystals confirms the diagnosis. This is true even without growth of the organism. It is our belief that a presumptive diagnosis of mycobacterial infection can be made if the clinical picture is typical, a granulomatous synovitis is identified histologically, rice bodies are found grossly, and examination for fungi and crystals are negative. Even without identification of acid-fast bacilli on special stains, antituberculous medication should be started immediately rather than waiting 4 to 8 weeks for growth of the organism.

TREATMENT

We believe that optimal treatment for mycobacterial infections is complete surgical synovectomy and early institution of antituberculous medications. There are a few reports in the literature of

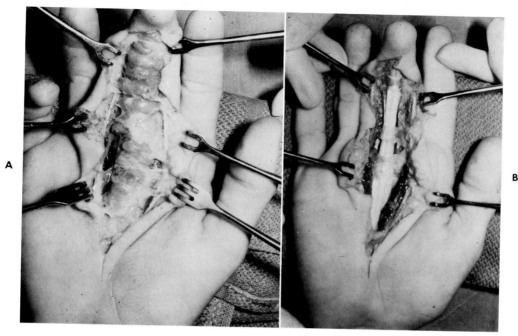

Fig. 8-23. A, A 17-year-old boy with a *Mycobacterium marinum* infection. **B,** Total synovectomy is done leaving the important flexor sheath pulleys, even though there may be some disease involvement.

cure from surgery alone[9] and from medications alone,[7] but there are the least complications with a combined program. In 4 of our 8 cases there has been wound breakdown and drainage after synovectomy. In three of these, the medications had not been started up to that point. The experience with *M. kansasii* pulmonary disease is that this organism is more sensitive than the others to the drugs. Unfortunately, one cannot be sure of the specific organism until nearly 6 weeks after biopsy, so it is impossible to know whether *M. kansasii* is the organism early in the treatment course. In Case 1, a presumptive diagnosis of *M. kansasii* was made based on the mode of injury, chronicity, and differential skin testing. However, that diagnosis was incorrect. We would have been much more comfortable with an initial complete synovectomy knowing that the organism was *M. marinum*. If this patient had reacted adversely to the antituberculous medications, requiring their discontinuation, he probably would not have been cured of his disease. There is enough poorly vascularized debris, such as rice bodies in the infected synovium, that it is reasonable to think that the drugs may not get to all the

infected tissue. Also, complete synovectomy allows earlier unencumbered motion in severe cases.

We have been satisfied with the zigzag incision for synovectomy. The exposure is excellent, and healing has been rapid. All of the involved disease should be removed with the exception that the annular pulleys must be saved (Fig. 8-23.). We prefer to save all four (Fig. 8-21, *C*), and we feel that at least the A2 and A4 pulleys must be kept. We would rather leave a partially infected but functioning pulley than remove all the pulleys and have to reconstruct them in a later surgical procedure. This certainly applies to *M. marinum, M. kansasii,* and *M. tuberculosis,* all of which will respond to drugs. In some cases of infections with Group III organisms, such as in Case 2, it may be necessary to excise all infected tissue.

The most effective drug regimen is isoniazid, ethambutol, and rifampin. It is very important that these be started as soon as the presumptive diagnosis is made as was done in Case 1. We feel that the drugs should be used in Group III infections as well, even though in vitro sensitivity testing usually shows resistance. The drugs should be continued for 18 to 24 months as they are in the treatment of pulmonary disease. It is quite possible that shorter periods would suffice in conjunction with surgical synovectomy, but this is not really known at this time.

REFERENCES

1. Cortez, L. M., and Pankey, G. A.: *Mycobacterium marinum* infections of the hand, J. Bone Joint Surg. **55-A:**363, 1973.
2. DeHaven, K., Wilde, A., and O'Duffy, T.: Sporotrichosis arthritis and tenosynovitis. Report of a case cured by synovectomy and amphotericin B, J. Bone Joint Surg. **54-A:**874, 1972.
3. Gunther, S. F.: Unpublished data.
4. Gunther, S., and Elliott, R.: *Mycobacterium kansasii* infection in the deep structures of the hand. Report of two cases, J. Bone Joint Surg. **58-A:**140, 1976.
5. Gunther, S., Elliott, R., Brand, R., and Adams, J.: Experience with atypical mycobacterial infection in the deep structures of the hand, J. Hand Surg. **2:**90, Mar., 1977.
6. Iverson, P., and Vistnes, L.: Coccidioidomycosis tenosynovitis in the hand, J. Bone Joint Surg. **55-A:**413, 1973.
7. Kaplan, M., and Clayton, M.: Carpal tunnel syndrome secondary to *Mycobacterium kansasii* infection, J.A.M.A. **208:**1186, 1969.
8. Kelly, P., Karlson, A., Weed, L., et al.: Infection of synovial tissues by mycobacteria other than *Mycobacterium tuberculosis*, J. Bone Joint Surg. **49-A:**1593, 1967.
9. Kelly, P. J., Weed, L. A., and Lipscomb, P. R.: Infection of tendon sheaths, bursae, joints, and soft tissues by acid-fast bacilli other than tubercle bacilli, J. Bone Joint Surg. **45-A:**327, 1963.
10. Klinenberg, J., Grimley, P., and Seegmiller, J.: Destructive polyarthritis due to a photochromogenic mycobacterium, N. Engl. J. Med. **272:**190, 1965.
11. Runyon, E., Karlson, A., Kubica, G., et al. In Lenette, E., Spaulding, E., and Truant, J., editors: Manual of clinical microbiology, Washington, D.C., 1974, The American Society of Microbiology, pp. 148-174.
12. Williams, D. S., and Riordan, D. C.: *Mycobacterium marinum* (atypical acid-fast bacillus) infections of the hand, J. Bone Joint Surg. **55-A:**1042, 1973.
13. Wolinsky, E.: Nontuberculous mycobacteria and associated diseases, Am. Rev. Resp. Dis. **119:**107, 1979.

Chapter 9

Principles of tendon transfers to the hand

RICHARD J. SMITH

HILL HASTINGS II

DEFINITION

In a *tendon transfer* a tendon is transected and reinserted into a bone or another tendon. The innervation and blood supply of its muscle are preserved. With a *tendon graft* a tendon is transected proximally and distally and is moved from one site to another without preserving its muscle or its vasculature. With a *free muscle transfer* a muscle/tendon is transected at its origin and insertion. The neurovascular stalk of the muscle is transected; after transfer the muscle is revascularized by appropriate vessel anastomosis, and neurorrhaphy is performed. Most often, a free muscle transfer is moved from one limb to another.

HISTORY

In the last half of the nineteenth century and in the early years of the twentieth century the techniques and principles of tendon transfer varied widely throughout the clinics of North America and Europe. Drobnik[31] lengthened tendons artificially with the use of silk strands. Vulpius[124] and Nicoladoni[85,86] sutured the tendon transfer into the paralyzed tendon rather than into bone. Lange[60] suggested that tendon transfers should be sutured with the greatest possible tension. Vulpius[123] recommended moderate tension. Stoffel[110] thought that there should be no tension at all.

The ideal bed for a tendon transfer was also the subject of dispute. Some thought the tendon should be drawn through subcutaneous tissue.[7,60] Others advocated a subfascial route.[124] Bunnell[19] transferred fatty tissues to the tendon bed.

In 1916 Mayer[71-74] published "The Physiological Method of Tendon Transplantation," based upon the results of his studies in the laboratories and clinics of Professor Biesalski[6] of Berlin. Mayer defined the following principles of tendon transfer, which remain the basis of our techniques:

1. A normal relationship should be reestablished between a transferred tendon and its sheath.
2. Tendon transfers should be sutured with no tension.
3. At surgery the limb should be positioned with minimal distance between the origin and insertion of the transfer.

In the years that followed, considerable attention was directed to methods of preventing adhesions around tendon transfers and grafts. Steindler[102] emphasized the importance of preserving the blood supply of the transfer. Bunnell and Boyes[19,20] clarified the principles of tendon transfer and demanded strict atraumatic technique. Surgeons inserted biologic interpositional membranes,* celloidin tubes,[75] stainless steel rods,[77,113] and flexible plastic implants† in order to form a sheath through which a tendon could glide. Investigation continues in the search for a reliable method of preventing adhesions, an effective tendon substitute, and a better understanding of physiology, anatomy, and biomechanics as they relate to tendon function.‡

---

*See references 1, 2, 5, 26, 40, 47, 48, 52, 53, 84, and 117.
†See references 3, 50, 55-57, and 96.
‡See references 28, 29, 39, 67, 70, 76, 87, 90, 91, and 119.

129

INDICATIONS
Substitution for the function of a paralyzed muscle

When disability results from irreversible paralysis due to neurological disease or nerve injury, the uninvolved muscles may be transferred to replace the function of the paralyzed muscles and to balance the forces around the limb.

If paralysis is due to peripheral nerve injury, the surgeon may choose to reconstruct the limb either by repairing the injured nerve, by tendon transfer, or by both neurorrhaphy and transfer. Neurorrhaphy is preferred if there is likelihood of muscle reinnervation as in younger patients if the injury is sharp and the nerve is repaired promptly.[97] In an older patient, if there has been crushing or traction on the injured nerve and if repair is delayed more than 6 months, the chance of restoring useful muscle recovery is less certain and early tendon transfer may be warranted. Pure motor nerves such as the radial nerve in the upper forearm recover more completely and reliably than do mixed nerves. Proximal muscles recover more completely than distal muscles.

After neurorrhaphy, axons may regrow at least 3 cm a month.[97] If we measure the distance from the site of nerve repair to the most proximal level of muscle innervation, we can calculate when to expect the earliest clinical and electrical signs of muscle recovery. If electromyography shows no signs of reinnervation after that time, one should consider appropriate reconstructive procedures, such as tendon transfer.

Omer[89] and Burkhalter[23] have suggested that a tendon transfer may serve as an *internal splint*. After severe injuries, tendon transfer and neurorrhaphy may be performed at the same operation. While the nerve is recovering, the transferred tendons enable the limb to function more normally, and they are "internal splints," which prevent joint contractures. For example, in an adult who recently suffered a median nerve injury caused by a bullet wound at the elbow, we would expect neurorrhaphy to result in reinnervation of the extrinsic muscles of the hand and restoration of sensibility to the fingers and thumb. However, we would not expect good thenar muscle recovery. If an opposition tendon transfer (opponensplasty) were performed at the time of neurorrhaphy, there would be useful thumb function while the nerve was regenerating. There would be little risk of adduction contracture or overcorrection even if some thenar function recovered.

Replacement of ruptured or avulsed tendons or muscles

Patients with rheumatoid disease of the hand may suffer tendon rupture because of ischemia,[80] synovial invasion,[111,112] or attrition of the tendon over bony spurs.* With severe injuries to the upper limb, tendons and muscles may be avulsed from the forearm and hand. If the muscle of a ruptured or avulsed tendon has retained its innervation and blood supply, a tendon graft can span the gap between the muscle and its insertion.[79,81] Residual forces are merely *redistributed* around a limb by tendon transfer; these forces are *restored* to a limb after successful tendon graft.

However, even if the muscle of an avulsed or ruptured tendon retains contractility, there may be advantages in replacing it by transfer rather than by graft. Although a tendon graft is avascular and must reestablish a blood supply throughout its length,[11,28] a tendon transfer retains the vessels entering the tendon from its musculocutaneous juncture.[28] A tendon graft is sutured proximally and distally; the transfer is sutured only at its distal end. For these reasons adhesions are more likely to develop around a graft than around a transfer.[36] If a tendon ruptured many months previously, its muscle may have become contracted and atrophied and lost much of its potential force and excursion. For this reason, when a patient with an old injury is treated, a transfer may be preferred to a tendon graft, since the donor muscle is functioning up to the day of operation.

In choosing between a tendon graft and a tendon transfer in the treatment of a patient with an avulsed or ruptured tendon, one must consider the quality of available donors, the length of time since injury, and the nature of the tendon bed.[101]

Restoration of balance to a deformed hand

In patients with cerebral palsy or other central nervous system disorders, some muscles may be spastic, while others may be weak. In most of these patients surgery is not indicated.[42,43,49] Sensibility of the hand, emotional, functional, and social factors, as well as the changing patterns of deformity, must be considered carefully before operation is planned. Occasionally, deformities caused by muscle imbalance may be corrected by appropriate tendon transfers.[106,107] Tight, spastic muscles are released and used to augment weaker

---

*See references 32, 45, 69, and 120-122.

muscles on the other side of the limb.[98] Tenotomy, tendon lengthening, and muscle slide procedures may be used in conjunction with tendon transfers.[99] Tenodesis, capsulodesis, and wrist fusion also must be considered.[106] Treatment of the hand in cerebral palsy is a field of special study and will not be considered here.

PREREQUISITES

In planning surgical reconstruction of the hand, the surgeon must know the functional and aesthetic goals of the patient. The patient must understand what to expect from the operation and what its limitations may be and be willing and able to cooperate in a program of postoperative care, which often includes further operative stages.

Tendon transfers are delayed until all inflammation and swelling have subsided, until joint contractures are freed by appropriate conservative and surgical care, and until a stable bony framework has been established. The bed through which the tendons will glide should be supple and soft. A tendon does not move through a vacuum, and the tissues that surround the transfer must be able to move with it. Free skin grafts and hypertrophic skin scar are not suitable covering for a tendon transfer and should be replaced by appropriate local or distant flaps before a tendon is transferred beneath it. A silicone rod may prepare a smooth bed for a tendon transfer.[75,78,101] If tendons are transferred prematurely, the results of the operation are jeopardized.

PRINCIPLES OF DONOR SELECTION

In selecting the appropriate muscle/tendon for transfer, we must choose a donor that is both functional and expendable. It must have adequate strength and amplitude. It is best if the transferred tendon travels a straight route and performs only one function. Postoperatively the muscle/tendon must be able to contract and relax appropriately to participate in smoothly integrated hand function. Critical hand function must not be lost by the transfer of the donor muscle/tendon.

Strength. The terms *force, work,* and *power* have been defined clearly by the physicist. *Force* is mass multiplied by acceleration.[104,108] Physicists measure force in terms of newtons, dynes, or pounds. Because the kilogram is a unit of mass, it should not be used to measure force. Clinically,

however a "kilogram of force" has been used in medical literature and is equal to pounds of force divided by 2.2. A dynamometer or pinchmeter is used clinically to measure the force exerted by the muscles that compress it.

The *force of a muscle is directly proportional to the cross-sectional area of all its muscle fibers* (Fig. 9-1). This is known as its *physiological cross section*. It has been calculated by Weber and Fick* that a muscle can exert a force of 3.6 kg per square centimeter or 50 lb per square inch of its physiologic cross-sectional area. Blix[8] found that the greatest force of contraction can be exerted when the muscle is at its resting length (Fig. 9-2). The force exerted by a muscle contraction decreases if the muscle fiber is further shortened or lengthened. The *viscoelastic force* of a muscle consists of the combined resistance to stretch produced by its muscle cells, fascia, and connective tissue.[98] Although the viscoelastic force of a muscle increases when it is stretched, the force of its contraction is *not* increased with stretching from the resting length (Fig. 9-3).

Work is force multiplied by distance.[34] With an isometric muscle contraction no work is performed, since the force exerted by the muscle does not move the limb. Similarly, if a muscle shortens or lengthens without being loaded, it has performed no work, since there is movement without force. The work capacity of a muscle is dependent both upon its physiologic cross section *and* the length of its muscle fibers, since work is the product of force and distance. Thus the work capacity of a given muscle is proportional to its mass[34] (Fig. 9-1). For example, the mass or volume of the flexor digitorum profundus and sublimis of the four fingers is seven times that of the mass or volume of the interossei and lumbricales combined.[15] Yet, the physiologic cross-sectional area of the extrinsics is only twice that of the intrinsics.[15] The work capacity of the extrinsics is therefore seven times that of the intrinsics. The amount of force that can be exerted by the extrinsics, however, is only twice that of the intrinsics.

Power is work per unit time. Thus, if a 10 kg mass is moved 10 cm in 1 second, twice the power is expended than if the same mass were moved the same distance in 2 seconds.

Clinicians frequently will use the terms force, work, power, and strength interchangeably. They will refer to the force exerted on a dynamom-

---

*See references 34, 35, 61, 108, and 116.

eter as "power" or "strength" of grip. Because these terms are accepted in the medical literature, we will use the term "strength" in its clinical sense to mean the force capacity of a muscle. We apologize to the bioengineer and the physicist who may, with good reason, object to the apparent misuse of these scientific terms.

The mass of each of the muscles of the forearm and hand is variable and depends upon the patient's sex, occupation, age, and general physical condition. However, the relative mass and physiologic cross section of each muscle in a normal limb remain relatively constant.[15] The following list of the comparative cross-sectional area and potential force of some of the muscles of the forearm and hand represents an approximation and extrapolation of studies by several authors[9,15,59,61]:

Muscle	Potential force
Brachioradialis	2.0
Flexor carpi ulnaris	2.0
FCR, ECRL, ECRB, ECU, PT, FPL, FDS, and FDP	1.0 (each tendon)
EDC, EIP, and EDQ	0.5 (each tendon)
APL, EPB, and PL	0.1 (each tendon)
Interossei	2.7 (total/combined)
Lumbricals	0.5 (total/combined)

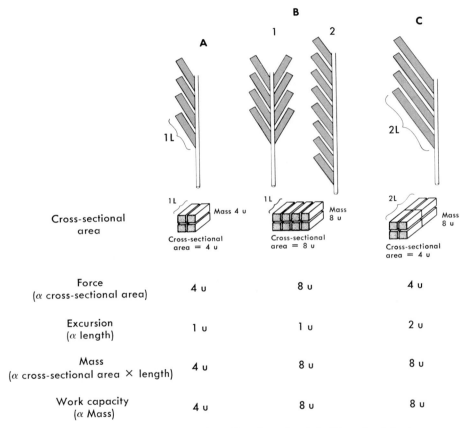

Fig. 9-1. A, A unipennate muscle with a fiber length of 1. The physiologic cross-sectional area as diagrammed is 4. Amplitude is proportional to its fiber length of 1. Potential force of the muscle is proportional to its cross-sectional area of 4. Work capacity is proportional to the mass; the cross-sectional area (4) multiplied by the length (1) equals mass of 4. **B,** A bipennate and a unipennate muscle with fiber lengths equal to that of muscle in **A,** but with twice the cross-sectional area. The potential force of muscle in **B** is twice that of muscle in **A.** The amplitude of muscle in **B** is equal to the one in **A.** The work capacity of muscle in **B** is double muscle in **A. C,** Muscle with the same cross-sectional area as in **A** but twice its fiber length. Potential force of muscle in **C** is equal to muscle in **A** and half of muscle in **B.** Its work capacity is twice that of muscle in **A** and equal to that of muscle in **B.**

In order to select the muscle with the proper strength (potential force) to use as a donor in a tendon transfer, the surgeon should consider (1) function of the transfer, (2) strength of the antagonist, and (3) mobility of the joints.

Function of the transfer. Is the transfer for grasp or for positioning a part of the hand? If it is for grasp, greater strength is needed. For example, the adductor pollicis is a muscle of grasp. It strongly pulls the thumb to the side of the index finger for activities such as turning a key in a tight lock, tearing a cloth, or pulling a cork from a bottle. Although the thumb may be adducted by

transfer of the extensor indicis proprius (EIP), this muscle is too weak for effective grasp. To restore power pinch after an ulnar nerve injury, we should select a donor muscle of sufficient strength to replace the paralyzed adductor. A

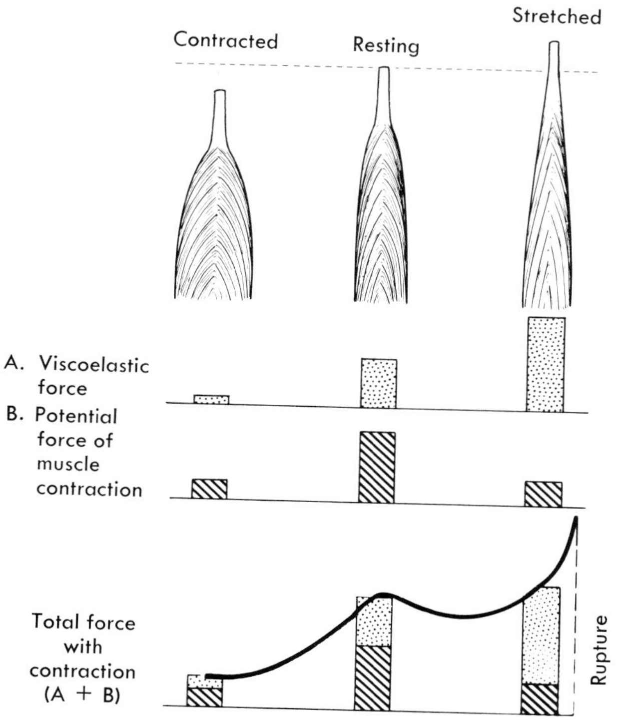

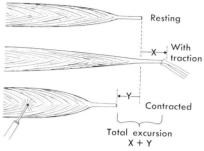

Fig. 9-3. A resting muscle can be stretched approximately 40% of its muscle fiber length. A muscle can contract approximately 40% of its muscle fiber length. The total excursion of a muscle is equal to the distance it can be stretched from its resting length *(X)* plus the distance it can contract from its resting length *(Y).*

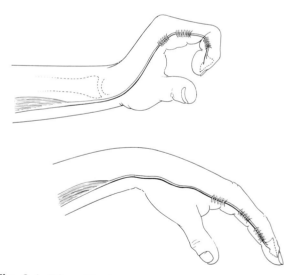

Fig. 9-2. The viscoelastic force of a muscle is increased as it is stretched to its breaking point. The potential force of muscle contraction, however, is greatest when the muscle is at its resting length. The potential force of muscle contraction decreases to zero when the resting muscle is either contracted 40% or stretched 40% of its fiber length. Although the potential force of a muscle contraction is greatest when the muscle is at resting length, the total force of a muscle equals the viscoelastic force plus the force of muscle contraction and gradually increases to the point of rupture.

Fig. 9-4. The effective amplitude of a muscle/tendon may be increased by the "tenodesis effect." Even without muscle contraction, dorsiflexing the wrist will cause the fingers to flex; palmarflexing the wrist will cause them to extend. This is due to the stretching and relaxation of the digital muscles/tendons as they cross the wrist joint. Absolute excursion of a muscle may be effectively increased if active motion of the intercalary joints is maintained.

wrist extensor or brachioradialis would have suitable strength. In contrast to the adductor, the thenar muscles are positioning muscles. Any transfer strong enough to lift the thumb into abduction would have sufficient strength to restore satisfactory opposition after thenar paralysis. Although the EIP would have insufficient strength to replace a paralyzed thumb adductor, it would have adequate strength to replace paralyzed thenar muscles.

Strength of the antagonist. When planning a tendon transfer, one must avoid overcorrection. For example, if the brachioradialis is used to replace a paralyzed thumb adductor in a patient who has transected the median and ulnar nerves at the wrist, the thumb may remain adducted against the side of the palm unless a strong abductor transfer is also performed. Suitable donors may not be available. Tendon transfers should be carefully selected in order to balance the potential force on either side of the paralyzed digit.

Mobility of joints. If a joint is hypermobile due to congenital joint laxity or prolonged paralysis, the surgeon must take particular care to avoid overcorrection. For example, to correct a paralytic clawhand, transfer of the flexor digitorum superficialis to the lateral bands may create a swan-neck deformity if the proximal interphalangeal joints are hypermobile. Another donor may be preferable.

Amplitude. The potential amplitude of a muscle is directly related to the resting length of its fibers.[34] The greatest potential force of contraction occurs when the fibers are at their resting length[8] (Fig. 9-4). The potential force of contraction decreases as its fibers shorten or are stretched. Once the muscle fibers have contracted 40% of their resting length, no additional force can be exerted. The amplitude of a muscle can be determined at operation. Traction upon a tendon will permit the surgeon to measure the length to which the resting muscle can be stretched by its antagonists. Usually this is approximately half the total amplitude of the muscle/tendon and 40% of its resting fiber length.[37] If the resting muscle is stimulated by faradic current, the distance through which its contracts, added to the distance through which the resting muscle can be stretched, equals the total absolute amplitude of the muscle/tendon.[37,88] The approximate excursion of muscles in the adult forearm and hand is as follows[9,15,59]:

BR	4.0 cm
FDP	7.0 cm
FDS	6.5 cm
EPL	6.0 cm
EDC and EIP	5.0 cm
FPL	5.0 cm
FCU, FCR, ECRL, ECRB, and ECU	3.0 cm
EPB and APL	3.0 cm
Lumbricals	3.8 cm
Thenars	3.8 cm
Interossei	2.0 cm

The "effective amplitude" or "relative amplitude" of a tendon transfer can be increased over that of the "absolute amplitude" by changing the position of the intercalary joints over which it passes. For example, if a wrist flexor (3 cm amplitude) is transferred to a finger flexor (7 cm amplitude), excellent active range of motion may be achieved if the wrist is mobile.[9,30,63] When the wrist is dorsiflexed, the "tenodesis effect" or stretching of the transfer added to the muscle contraction will increase the effective amplitude of the transferred wrist flexor (Fig. 9-4). Wrist motion may increase the effective amplitude of a muscle by 25 to 30 mm.

Effective amplitude of a muscle/tendon may also be increased by freeing the soft tissues that limit muscle contraction. For example, amplitude of the brachioradialis can be increased 20 to 45 mm by freeing the fascia that surrounds the muscle and tendon.[9,37]

Direction. A tendon transfer should, if possible, pass in a straight line from its origin to its insertion. If a tendon transfer must change direction during its course, it should be passed around a stable, smooth, and ample pulley. A Y juncture is formed if a donor tendon is transferred to the recipient tendon that remains with its paralyzed muscle. A Y juncture may divert the direction of the transfer. For this reason we will transect the recipient tendon proximal to the site of suture (Fig. 9-5).

Integrity. A tendon transfer should have only one function. However, it may be inserted into more than one recipient. For example, FCU may be transferred to the extensors of all five digits. FDS may be transferred to the dorsal aponeurosis of two fingers. In each case the transfer performs a similar function in several digits. By contrast, in a patient with a low ulnar nerve palsy if a tendon is split and transferred both to adduct the

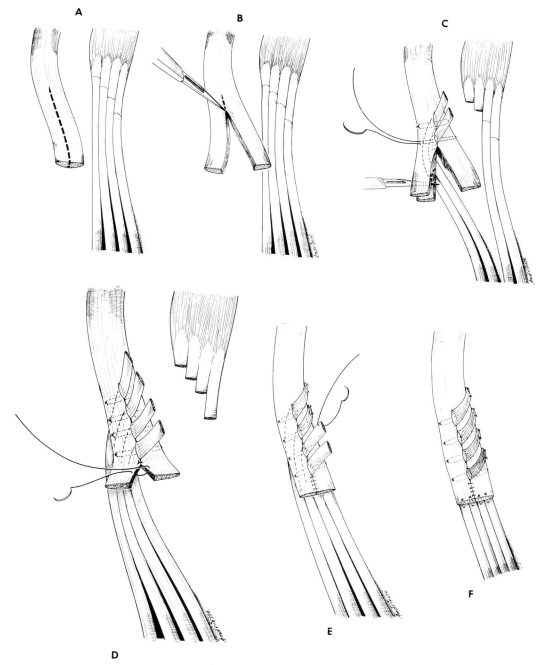

Fig. 9-5. One means of joining a tendon donor to multiple tendon recipients is by the "sandwich suture." **A** and **B,** The donor tendon is split longitudinally. **C,** The recipient tendons are transected, and each tendon is fixed to the donor tendon with horizontal mattress sutures. The distal end of the donor tendon is thinned. **D,** After all recipient tendons have been sutured to the donor tendon, the distal end of the donor is closed. **E,** The proximal ends of the recipient tendons are sutured to the side of the donor tendon. **F,** The distal end of the donor tendon is sutured to the recipient tendons. This method allows adjustment of the length of each tendon and provides a secure juncture. Donor and recipient muscles do not form a Y with the recipient tendon.

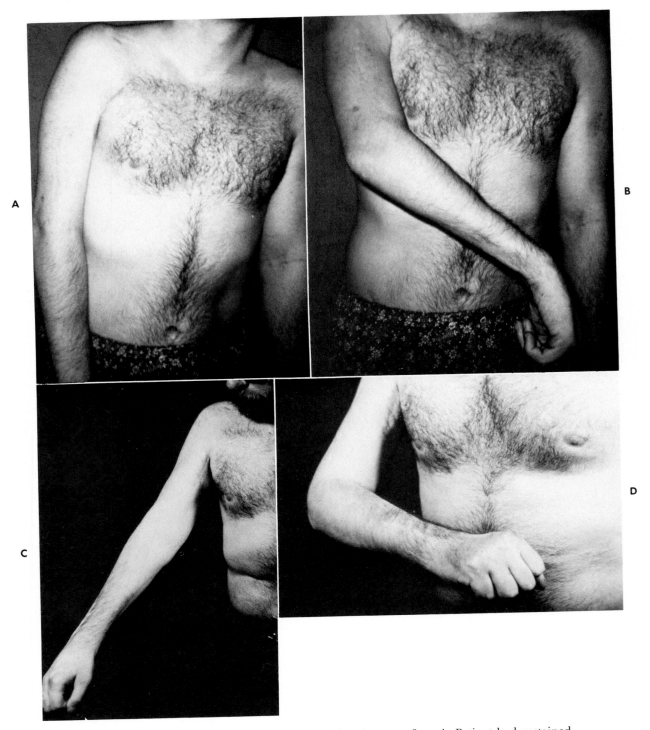

Fig. 9-6. Restoration of "integrity" to muscle/tendon transfers. **A,** Patient had sustained multiple injuries to his upper limb, including loss of elbow flexion and wrist extension. A Steindler flexorplasty was performed, moving the origin of the wrist flexors and pronators of the forearm to the anterior aspect of the distal humerus. **B,** When he attempts to bend the elbow, the flexor-pronator group flexes both the forearm and the wrist. The muscles were performing two functions poorly. They did not have "integrity" of function. **C** and **D,** Subsequent to wrist arthrodesis, the flexor-pronator transfer had but one function: elbow flexion. The elbow now flexes strongly through 70 degrees.

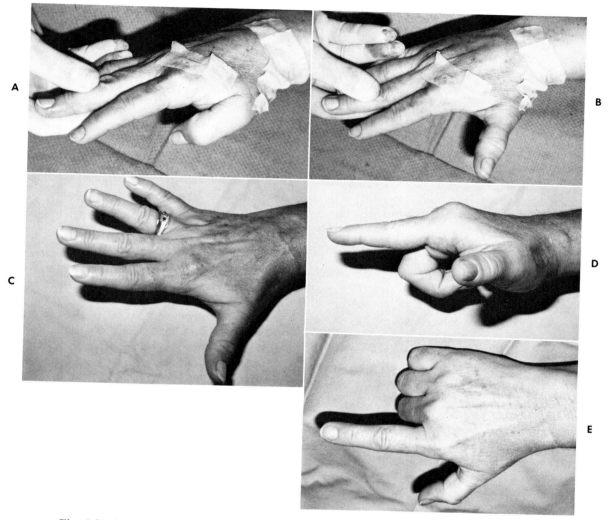

Fig. 9-7. A, Immediately following a transfer of extensor indicis proprius to replace a ruptured extensor pollicis longus, the patient's thumb remains partially flexed. **B,** The patient is asked to extend the thumb. She spontaneously contracts the transferred extensor indicis proprius for thumb IP extension. Both visual clues and proprioceptive feedback permit immediate use of the index extensor for its new function. No retraining was necessary. **C,** Two months later the transferred tendon is used spontaneously, smoothly, and unconsciously. **D,** Patient can extend the index finger independently of the other fingers. **E,** Simultaneous flexion of the IP joint of the thumb and extension of the index finger is possible through selective contraction of the index extensor communis and relaxation of the extensor indicis proprius. No "relearning" was necessary.

thumb and to flex the metacarpophalangeal (MP) joints of the fingers, it may not succeed. The excursion, power, and direction required of the two recipients are different. The transfer may not perform both functions effectively.

The integrity of a transfer also may be compro-

mised if it crosses several joints that are not under active control. For example, in patients with biceps and brachialis paralysis following musculocutaneous nerve loss, we can restore elbow flexion by transfer of the origin of the flexor-pronator muscles of the forearm from the medial epicondyle to the shaft of the humerus.[105,106] This transfer increases the moment arm of the flexor-pronator group at the elbow. The operation is known as the *Steindler flexorplasty*. If the transfer is performed in a patient who also has a radial nerve palsy, the flexor-pronator muscles will flex both the elbow and the wrist simultaneously, and the integrity of the transfer is lost. The amplitude of the transfer will be divided between the two joints, and neither elbow flexion nor wrist flexion will be satisfactory. If the wrist is then arthrodesed, integrity is restored, and elbow flexion is regained (Fig. 9-6).

Synergy. Should synergistic muscles be chosen as donors in tendon transfers? *Synergistic* muscles are those which work together to move a joint. Muscles that have an opposite action on a joint are considered *antagonistic*. Yet antagonists may work together, and synergists may not. The extensor carpi radialis longus (ECRL) and flexor carpi ulnaris (FCU) are antagonists. They have opposite action at the wrist: one extends and radially deviates; the other flexes and ulnarly deviates. Yet when we hammer a nail, both muscles work together (in synergy?), controlling the force and speed with which the nail is struck and the hammer elevated. The EPL and the thenar muscles are synergistic. They both extend the distal joint of the thumb. Yet the thenars extend the thumbtip only when the MP joint is flexed and the thumb is in opposition; the EPL contracts only when the MP joint and the interphalangeal (IP) joint are to be extended. Thus muscles that have the same insertion may not work together.

Motor skills are not learned as a sequence of muscle contractions to be programmed like the roll in a player piano. Rather, the brain recruits the best muscles available to do the job. The sensory cortex evaluates how well the job is being performed. If some muscles are unable to achieve the proper function, the brain will recruit substitutes. If a man writes his signature 6 inches high on a blackboard, his normal handwriting changes little. Yet he is using muscles totally different from those he usually uses when he is comfortably seated and writing his name on a piece of paper. When he attempts to write with his eyes closed, his handwriting changes appreciably. If the loss of visual feedback is compounded by a loss of sensory feedback as with peripheral nerve injury or cerebral palsy, handwriting becomes illegible.

Electromyograms performed after tendon transfers have shown that muscles will contract appropriately to their new position within one day of the operation.[62] We do not need to instruct the patient how to use the tendon transfer. We need only to encourage him to use his hands. The transfer will contract in its new phase for its new function.

In most cases, synergy does not appear to be crucial in selecting appropriate muscles for transfer (Fig. 9-7).

METHOD OF DONOR SELECTION

The best plan for surgical reconstruction of a limb with paralysis or tendon loss will depend upon the donors available, the nature and extent of the disability, and the function we hope to restore. The following method of planning a surgical program has been found useful:

Step 1: What works? Make a "working" list of all muscles with fair, good, or excellent power.

Step 2: What's available? Make an "available" list of the "working" muscles that may be transferred. Be certain that after tendons are transferred there will remain at least one wrist flexor, one wrist extensor, and one flexor and extensor for each digit.

Step 3: What's needed? Make a "needed" list of those functions—not muscles—that are to be replaced.

Step 4: Matching. Match available muscles and needed function on the basis of the principles of tendon transfer considering the amplitude, power, direction, and integrity of the potential transfer.

Step 5: Alternatives. If all desired functions cannot be obtained by tendon transfer, consider the alternatives of capsulodesis, tenodesis, arthrodesis, or pully release.

Step 6: Staging. Divide the surgical procedures into three stages:
1. Transfers on the *flexor* side of the hand
2. Transfers on the *extensor* side of the hand.
3. Transfers passing both volar and dorsal to the joints of the hand

Some surgeons have recommended that the extensor transfers should precede the flexor transfers in treating patients with quadriplegia.

EXAMPLE OF METHOD OF DONOR SELECTION

A 24-year-old woman with quadriplegia has lost the function of her right hand. What reconstructive procedures would you advise?

Step 1: **What works?** Which muscles are fair or better? Muscle testing reveals that the functioning muscles include the following:

Working
BR
PT
ECRL
ECRB
ECU
FCU (fair)
FCR
PQ

Step 2: **What is available?** Since all three wrist extensors function well, two are available for transfer. We may use ECRL and extensor carpi ulnaris (ECU), allowing extensor carpi radialis brevis (ECRB) to remain for wrist extension. Both wrist flexors are available, but FCU is only "fair." Either FCU or flexor carpi radialis (FCR), but not both, may be transferred. There are two pronators; pronator teres (PT) is available. The following muscles are therefore selected for transfer:

Working	*Available*
BR	BR
PT	PT
ECRL	ECRL
ECRB	
ECU	ECU
FCU (fair)	FCU (fair)
FCR	
PQ	

Step 3: **What is needed?** We would like to have finger flexion, thumb flexion, finger extension, thumb extension, thumb opposition, MP flexion-IP extension (intrinsic function), and thumb adduction.

Working	*Available*	*Needed*
BR	BR	Finger flexion
PT	PT	Thumb flexion
ECRL	ECRL	Finger extension
ECRB		Thumb extension
ECU	ECU	Thumb opposition
FCU (fair)	FCU (fair)	MP flexion-IP extension
FCR		(intrinsics)
PQ		Thumb adduction

Step 4: **Matching.** Match columns 2 and 3 on the basis of principles of tendon transfer.

Working	*Available*	*Needed*
BR	BR →	Finger flexion
PT	PT →	Thumb flexion
ECRL	ECRL →	Finger extension
ECRB		Thumb extension
ECU	ECU and graft →	Thumb opposition
FCU (fair)	FCU (fair) →	MP flexion-IP extension
FCR		(intrinsics)
PQ	?? →	Thumb adduction

Continued.

EXAMPLE OF METHOD OF DONOR SELECTION—cont'd

Other operative plans could be considered. Arthrodesis of the wrist would permit all wrist extensors and flexors to be transferred, thereby adding two more donors. One of these donors could be used for thumb adduction. However, with the wrist arthrodesed, the patient would not benefit from a tenodesis effect of wrist motion, and full active finger motion probably would not be achieved. Some surgeons might prefer to restore thumb adduction rather than opposition in order to provide good keypinch. Others might choose to transfer a tendon to the abductor pollicis longus in order to stabilize the thumb base. The best plan is based on many factors including the patient's functional requirements, joint mobility, deformities of the limb, the nature of abnormalities of other limbs, and, to some extent, the experience of the surgeon.

Step 5: **Alternatives.** Is arthrodesis or tenodesis necessary? Good pinch may be achieved by thumb IP arthrodesis after brachioradialis (BR) transfer to the flexor pollicis longus (FPL). This would improve pulp-to-side pinch. We might thus consider thumb IP arthrodesis for stronger adduction.

Step 6: **Staging.** Divide surgical procedures into stages, according to whether postoperative immobilization will be in flexion or extension.

Available	Needed	Flexion or extension	Operative stage
BR ———————→	Thumb flexion	Flexion	First
PT ———————→	Finger extension	Extension	Second
	Thumb extension		
ECRL ———————→	Finger flexion	Flexion	First
ECU ———————→	Intrinsics	Both	Third
FCU ———————→	Thumb opposition	Flexion	First
(IP arthrodesis)	Thumb adduction	Neither	Second

Therefore, following would be our surgical plan:
Stage 1: BR to FPL; ECRL to FDP; FCU to EPB for thumb opposition.
Stage 2: PT to EPL and EDC; thumb IP arthrodesis.
Stage 3: ECU is prolonged with plantaris graft, routed volar to deep transverse metacarpal ligament, and sutured to lateral bands of index, middle, ring, and little fingers.

The patient will be instructed that at least three operations are necessary. She should anticipate a clenched fist after the first stage. She should anticipate a clawhand after the second stage. Hopefully, she will have a well-balanced hand after the third stage. Three to 6 months will be permitted between stages (Fig. 9-8).

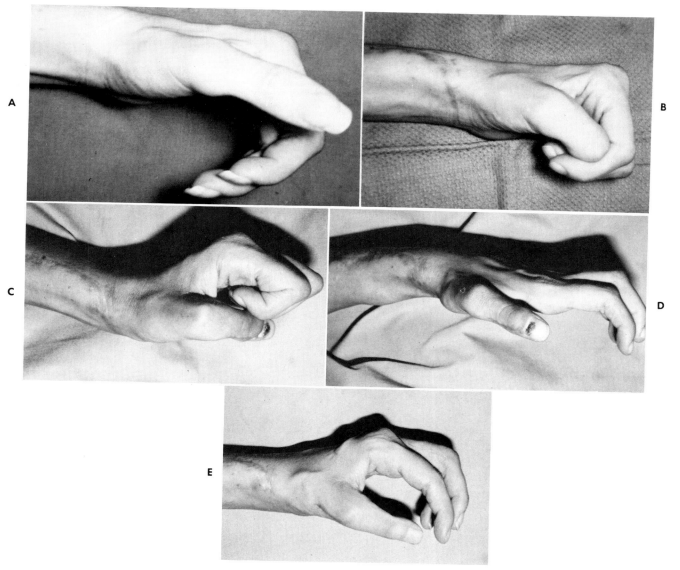

Fig. 9-8. A, A 24-year-old woman with quadriplegia lost function of her left hand. She had absent intrinsics and digital flexors and extensors, but good wrist and forearm muscles. **B,** Stage 1, flexors. Brachioradialis was transferred to FPL. ECRL was transferred to FDP. The fingers can now flex but cannot extend. **C** and **D,** Stage 2, extensors. Following transfer of pronator teres to EPL and EDC and arthrodesis of the IP joint of the thumb, she was able to flex and extend all digits **(C).** She now has developed clawing of the fingers and is still unable to oppose the thumb **(D). E,** Stage 3, intrinsics. Following intrinsic transfer (ECU prolonged with plantaris to the lateral bands) and opposition transfer (FCU prolonged by rerouted EPB to thumb proximal phalanx), balance of the hand is restored, and she is able to use the hand for activities of daily living.

TENDON TRANSFERS FOR ISOLATED NERVE INJURY

Many tendon transfers have been described for common patterns of paralysis. Most have successfully withstood the test of extensive clinical trial.

The choice of transfer must always be based on the defects and the needs of each patient. Some of the more popular tendon transfers are listed both for reference and for their historic value (Table 7).

Table 7. Tendon transfers

LOW MEDIAN NERVE PALSY—TRANSFERS FOR OPPOSITION[99]

Donor	Pulley	Graft	Insertion on thumb	Reference
FDS (ring)	Distal FCU	None	Dorsal-ulnar base PP	Bunnell, 1938[21]
FDS (ring)	FCU	None	APB	Littler, 1949[64]
FDS (ring)	FCU	None	APB and EPL at PP	Riordan, 1959[94]
FDS (ring)	Guyon canal	None	APB and EPL	Brand, 1966[13]
EIP	Ulnar side of wrist	None	PP	Zancolli, 1965[125] and 1968[126] Burkhalter, 1973[24] Fig. 9-9
ADQ	None	None	APB	Huber, 1921[54] Littler and Cooley, 1963[65]
PL	Carpal tunnel	Rerouted EPB	EPB	Ney, 1921[83]
PL	None	Palmar fascia	Radial side MPJ	Camitz, 1929[27] Littler, 1967[66]
Half FPL	Around radial side of thumb	None	Dorsal PP	Steindler, 1918[103]
FPL	Translocated dorsally	None	PP	Makin, 1967[68]
FPL	Transverse carpal ligament	None	PP and DP	Williams, 1966[118]
APL	PL	None	Base MC	Edgerton and Brand, 1965[33]
ECU	Ulnar side of wrist	Rerouted EPB	EPB	Phalen and Miller, 1947[92]
ECRL or ECRB	Ulnar side of wrist	Free graft	EPL	Henderson, 1962[51]

HIGH MEDIAN NERVE PALSY

Donor	Insertion	Function	Reference
EIP	APB	Opposition	Fig. 9-9
BR	FPL	Thumb flexion	Smith and Hastings, 1980 (unpublished)
Thumb IP arthrodesis		Thumb IP stability	
FDP (ring and little)	FDP (index and middle)	Finger flexion	
EIP	APB	Opposition	Burkhalter, 1974[23]
ECRL	FDP (index and middle)	Finger flexion	
BR	FPL	Thumb flexion	
FCU with graft	Thumb PP	Opposition	Goldner, 1974[46]
ECRL	FDP (index and middle)	Finger flexion	
BR	FPL	Thumb flexion	
Thumb IP arthrodesis		Thumb IP stability	
ECU with graft	Thumb PP	Opposition	Boyes, 1970[9]
BR	FDP (index and middle)	Finger flexion	
FDP (ring and little)			
ECRL or ECRB	FPL	Thumb flexion	

Continued.

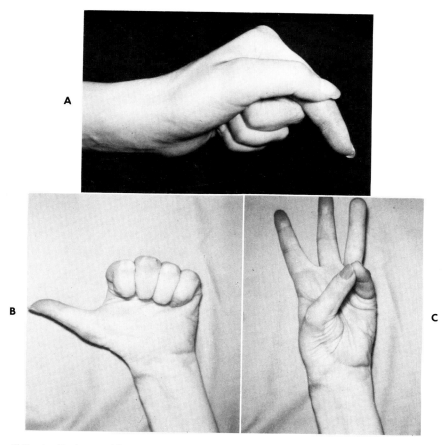

Fig. 9-9. A, Patient with a high median nerve palsy has no thumb or index finger flexion. There is weak flexion of the middle finger and no opposition. **B,** Operation included IP arthrodesis of the thumb, EIP transfer for opposition, and suture of the distal ends of flexor profundus of index and middle fingers to flexor profundus of the ring finger. Full finger flexion was restored. **C,** Patient regained good opposition of the thumb.

Table 7. Tendon transfers—cont'd

HIGH MEDIAN NERVE PALSY—cont'd

Donor	Insertion	Function	Reference
ECU with graft	Thumb PP	Opposition	Brand, 1975[14]
FDP (ring and little)	Sutured to FDP (index and middle)	Finger flexion	
ECRL	FPL	Thumb flexion	
FCU split	FCR and FCU	Wrist balance	

LOW ULNAR NERVE PALSY[104,108]
To correct clawing

Donor	Insertion	Reference
FDS	EDC	Stiles, 1922[109]
FDS (ring)	Radial lateral bands (index and middle)	Bunnell, 1942[22]
FDS (middle)	Radial lateral bands (ring and little)	
FCR with tendon graft	Lateral bands	Riordan, 1959[94]
EDQ and EIP	Lateral bands	Bunnell, 1942[19]; Fowler, 1946[94]
ECRB or ECRL with tendon graft	Lateral bands	Brand, 1961[10-12]
ECRL or BR with tendon graft	Proximal phalanx	Burkhalter, 1973[25]
FCR with tendon graft	Pulley (Lasso operation)	Brooks and Jones, 1974[16]
FDS	Pulley (Lasso operation)	Zancolli, 1974[127]
PL with tendon graft	Lateral bands	Fritschi, 1971[38]

To restore index abduction

Donor	Insertion	Reference
EIP	Tendon of first DI	Brown, 1974[17]
ECRL with graft	Tendon of first DI	Goldner, 1953[41]
EPB	Tendon of first DI	Bruner, 1948[18]; Littler, 1949[64]
EDQ	Tendon of first DI	Zweig, 1972[128]
FDS	Tendon of first DI	Goldner, 1953[41]; Littler, 1949[64]
APL (extra slip) with graft	Tendon of first DI	Neviaser, Wilson, and Gardner, 1980[82]

To restore thumb adduction

Donor	Route	Insertion	Reference
ECRB with graft	Between second and third metacarpal	Adductor pollicis	Smith and Hastings, 1980 (unpublished)
FDS	Between radius and ulna; around ECU	PP thumb	Goldner, 1967[44]
FDS	Across palm	Adductor pollicis and EPL	Tubiana, 1969[115]
FDS	Across palm	Adductor pollicis	Thompson, 1949[114]
FDS		Graft between base of thumb and fifth metacarpal	Bunnell, 1942[22]; Boyes, 1970[9]
EDC-index	Ulnar side wrist	Adductor pollicis	Bunnell, 1942[22]; Boyes, 1970[9]
BR or ECRL with graft	Between third and fourth metacarpal	Adductor pollicis	Boyes, 1970[9]
FDS (little)	Across palm	Adductor pollicis	Zancolli, 1968[126]
EPB	Through carpal canal	Adductor pollicis	Zancolli, 1968[126]
EDQ	Dorsum hand	Adductor pollicis and first dorsal IO	Zweig, Rosenthal, and Burns, 1972[128]

Table 7. Tendon transfers—cont'd

COMBINED MEDIAN AND ULNAR NERVE PALSY

Donor	Insertion	Function	Reference
ECU with FDS graft	Thumb PP	Thumb opposition	Goldner, 1974[45]
ECRL	FDP	Finger flexion	
BR	FPL	Thumb flexion	
Thumb IP fusion		Thumb IP stability	
EIP	First Dl	Index abduction	
MP volar capsulodeses		Correct clawing	
EPB rerouted volar around PL	Thumb PP	Thumb opposition	Brand, 1975[14]
ECRL	FDP	Finger flexion	
ECU	FPL	Thumb flexion	
Thumb IP fusion		Thumb IP stability	
EIP and EDQ	Lateral bands	Intrinsics	
FPL rerouted across thenar subcutaneously	Extensor mechanism at thumb MP joint	Thumb opposition	Riordan, 1964[95]
ECRL	FDP	Finger flexion	
ECU	FPL	Thumb flexion	
FCU with graft	APB	Thumb opposition	Littler, 1949[64]
ECRL	FDP	Finger flexion	
EDQ	FPL	Thumb flexion	
EPB	First D1	Index abduction	

HIGH RADIAL NERVE PALSY

Donor	Insertion	Function	Reference
PT	ECRL and ECRB	Wrist extension	Jones, 1921[58]
FCR	EPL, EPB, APL, and EDC (index)	Thumb extension, abduction, index extension	
FCU	EDC	Finger extension	
PT	ECRB	Wrist extension	Goldner, 1974[45]
FDS (middle)	EPL (rerouted)	Thumb extension and abduction	
FCU	EDC	Finger extension	
PT	ECRB	Wrist extension	Brand, 1975[14]
PL	EPL	Thumb extension	
FCR	EDC	Finger extension	
PT	ECRL and ECRB	Wrist extension	Boyes, 1970[9]
FCR	APL and EPB	Thumb abduction	
FDS (ring)	EPL and EIP	Thumb and index extension	
FDS (middle)	EDC	Finger extension	
PT	ECRL	Wrist extension	Riordan, 1964[95]
PL	EPL (rerouted)	Thumb extension and abduction	
FCU	EDC	Finger extension	
PT	ECRB	Wrist extension	Beasley, 1970[4]
PL	APL	Thumb abduction	
FDS (little)	EPL	Thumb extension	
FDS (ring)	EDC	Finger extension	
PT	ECRB	Wrist extension	Fig. 9-10
FCU	EDC and EPL	Digit extension	Smith and Hastings, 1980 (unpublished)

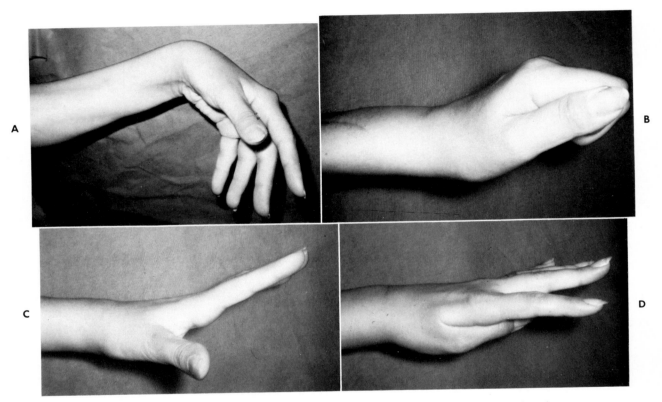

Fig. 9-10. A, Following removal of a large tumor of the upper arm, the patient has a permanent radial nerve palsy. **B,** Flexor carpi ulnaris was transferred to the extensors of the fingers and thumb. Pronator teres was transferred to the extensor carpi radialis brevis. Patient was able to actively dorsiflex the wrist 45 degrees. **C,** Finger and thumb extension are complete even with the wrist in neutral. **D,** Despite transfer of one donor to all digital extensors, patient is able to flex thumb while holding the fingers in extension.

POSTOPERATIVE CARE

A tendon transfer must be protected from abnormal tension until tendon juncture has united and the tendon has revascularized. Although maximum tensile strength of a tendon juncture is not achieved for at least 3 months, it is usually safe to begin active range of motion exercises after 3 to 4 weeks. We do not usually "retrain" transferred tendons. We do not suggest that the patient imitate the initial function of the donor tendon. Such "relearning" would be difficult under any circumstances and would be impossible after multiple tendon transfers. Rather, the patient is asked to move the hand actively and slowly through a full range of motion at all joints. The patient is given a schedule of manual activities that require the use of the tendon transfer and is asked to perform these activities several times a day. The help of the occupational, physical, or hand therapist is often valuable. For an additional 3 to 6 weeks, a protective splint is worn at all times when the hand is most subject to accidental force such as when the patient is sleeping, outdoors, at work, or around children. In special circumstances such as with tendon transfers in patients with cerebral palsy or arthrogryposis, we may continue the use of a protective splint for up to 6 months.

SPECIFIC TECHNICAL PROBLEMS

Among the more difficult technical problems that must be solved when performing tendon transfers is how to determine the proper length of the tendon transfer. Mayer[72-74] has established the rule that the transfer should be sutured under no tension at its resting length. He also suggested that the transfer should be sutured so that the origin of the donor muscle is closest to the insertion of the recipient tendon. In many cases this may lead to overcorrection of upper limb deformities.[37] What, then, is the proper length of the transfer?

The length at which a tendon transfer is sutured depends on the comparative amplitude of the donor and the recipient, the comparative power of the donor and its antagonist, and the function of the recipient. For example, if the antagonist is weak (as with an opposition transfer in a patient with combined low ulnar and median nerve palsy), the transfer is made slightly longer. If the antagonist is strong (FCU to ECRL in a pa-

tient with cerebral palsy and a spastic FCR), the transfer is sutured slightly shorter, with no tension but with the limb placed in full correction when the tendon is sutured. If the transfer is to function for prehension such as ECRL to flexor digitorum profundus (FDP), it is made shorter. If it is for positioning such as FCU to extensor digitorum communis (EDC), it is made longer. Despite the excursion or power of the transfer, the surgeon should be able to move all intercalary joints through a full range of motion after the transfer is sutured in place. For example, if the wrist cannot be fully palmar flexed after a transfer for finger extension, the transfer is too short and should be lengthened.

With several available donors of similar strength, amplitude, and direction, which should be chosen? The experience and preference of surgeons varies. Following are our preferences for donor muscles.

Flexor digitorum superficialis (FDS). We will use FDS of the middle and ring fingers as donors but will transect the tendons opposite the neck of the proximal phalanx to permit the distal FDS stump to become adherent to the volar plate. This helps to prevent secondary swan-neck deformity of the donor finger. When using FDS to restore intrinsic muscle function with an isolated low ulnar nerve palsy, the middle finger is used as the donor to avoid swan-neck deformity in the recipient fingers. We have occasionally seen FDS work "out of phase" when it is transferred to the EDC. In these patients we have actively retrained the transfers to work "in phase" by electrical stimulation of the FDS while the patient attempted finger extension. In no other instance have we found it necessary to "retrain" muscles. We will rarely use FDS of the index finger for a donor because it is too important for index pinch. We rarely use FDS of the little finger as a donor because it is often quite weak and may arise from a common muscle shared with FDS of the ring finger.

Wrist flexors. If the FCR and the FCU are both available for transfer, we will usually choose FCR as the donor in the manual worker. This preserves strong wrist flexion in ulnar deviation, which is important for activities such as chopping, cutting, and using a screwdriver or pliers. With more extensive paralysis, where the patient will not return to manual work, we prefer trans-

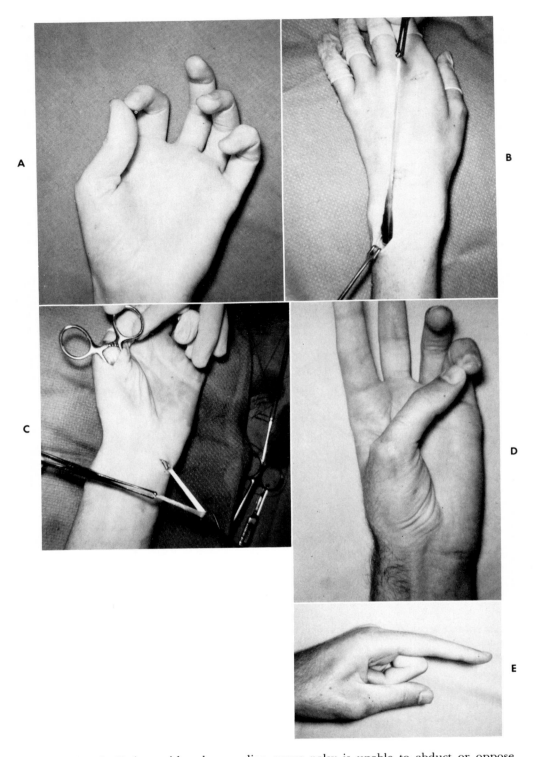

Fig. 9-11. A, Patient with a low median nerve palsy is unable to abduct or oppose thumb. **B,** Extensor indicis proprius is transected at its insertion and freed to the distal third of the forearm. **C,** Extensor indicis proprius is transferred anteriorly and passed through a subcutaneous tunnel to the radial base of the thumb proximal phalanx. **D,** Abduction and pronation are restored. **E,** Patient retains ability to extend the index finger independently, since the extensor communis is not tethered to the adjacent extensors by juncturae tendinum.

fer of the FCU. The wrist will then palmar flex in the straight AP plane, increasing the tenodesis effect upon the digital extensors.

Wrist extensors. ECRB is the most effective wrist extensor. ECRL and ECU each dorsiflex the wrist and deviate the hand away from its sagittal axis. However, when ECRL and ECU contract simultaneously, the wrist dorsiflexes without deviating medially or laterally. For this reason, if only one of the extensors is needed for transfer, we will choose the ECRB. Postoperatively, the patient will be able to dorsiflex the wrist in neutral or in radial or ulnar deviation. If two donors are necessary, we will choose the ECRL and ECU.

Brachioradialis. Brachioradialis (BR) is a powerful muscle. Its excursion can be increased by freeing it to the proximal forearm. A rather long forearm incision is therefore necessary if BR is to be used as the donor.

Extensor indicis proprius (EIP). EIP is an excellent donor tendon for thumb or finger extension or for thumb opposition. We have found the index finger continues to extend independently at the metacarpophalangeal joint after the EIP has been transferred. (See Figs. 9-7 and 9-11.) Independent index extension is preserved, since the index extensor digitorum communis (EDC) is not connected to its neighbors by junctura tendinae.

Extensor digiti quinti (EDQ). In many normal hands the EDC has only a small slip to the little finger. EDQ is the principal MP extensor in these hands. For this reason we will avoid using the EDQ as a transfer if other suitable tendons are available.

Free muscle transfers. With recent advances in microsurgery free muscle transfers have proven an effective means of restoring function to injured limbs. To date the experience with free muscle transfers is limited. However, it seems certain that they will prove a valuable means of treating patients with Volkmann's contracture and severe soft tissue loss of the forearm and hand. Today these transfers have only limited application in patients with isolated injury or paralysis.

CONCLUSIONS

Poliomyelitis is rare throughout most of the world. Leprosy can now be treated successfully. Advances in surgical techniques have greatly improved the results of neurorrhaphy. Yet, our hospital beds remain filled with patients with ir-

reversible paralysis. Farm and factory machines, the automobile, and the motorcycle have replaced infectious diseases as a major cause of serious musculoskeletal disability. Injuries that would have been fatal years ago now leave victims with irreparable lesions of the spinal cord, brachial plexus, or peripheral nerves. With expert primary care these patients often can anticipate a normal life span. With effective reconstructive surgery they can also look forward to a productive, meaningful life-style.

A versatile hand is one with balance, mobility, and strength. Tendon transfers are often the means by which the paralyzed or severely injured limb can regain this versatility.

REFERENCES

1. Ashley, F. L., Polak, T., Stone, R. S., and Marmor, L.: Healing of tendons in silicone rubber sheaths, Bull. Dow-Corning **4**:3, 1962.
2. Ashley, F. L., Stone, R. S., Alonso-Artieda, M., Syverud, J. M., Edwards, J. W., and Mooney, S. A.: Experimental and clinical studies on the application of monomolecular cellulose filter tubes to create artificial tendon sheaths in digits, Plast. Reconstr. Surg. **23**:526, 1959.
3. Bassett, C. A., and Carroll, R. E.: Formation of tendon sheath by silicone rod implants, J. Bone Joint Surg. **45-A**:884, 1963.
4. Beasley, R. W.: Tendon transfers for radial nerve palsy, Orthop. Clin. North Am. **2**:439, 1970.
5. Biesalski, K.: Ueber Sehnenscheidenauswechslung, Dtsch. Med. Wochnschr. **36**:1615, 1910.
6. Biesalski, K., and Mayer, L.: Die physiologische sehneneurphanzung, Berlin, 1916, Julius Springer.
7. Billington, R. W.: Tendon transplantation for musculospiral (radial) nerve injury, J. Bone Joint Surg. **4**:538, 1922.
8. Blix, M.: Die lange und die spannung des muskels, Skandinaviches Arch. F. Physiol. **3**:295, 1891; **4**:399, 1893; **5**:150, 1894.
9. Boyes, J. H., editor: Bunnell's surgery of the hand, ed. 5, Philadelphia, 1970, J. B. Lippincott Co.
10. Brand, P. W.: Paralytic clawhand with special reference to paralysis in leprosy and treatment by the sublimus transfer of Stiles and Bunnell, J. Bone Joint Surg. **40-B**:618, 1958.
11. Brand, P. W.: Tendon grafting illustrated by a new operation for intrinsic paralysis of the fingers, J. Bone Joint Surg. **43-B**:444, 1961.
12. Brand, P. W.: Deformity in leprosy. In Cochrane, R. G., and Devey, T. F., editors: Leprosy in theory and practice, ed. 2, Bristol, England, 1964, Wright and Sons, Ltd., pp. 447-492.
13. Brand, P. W.: The hand in leprosy. In Pulvertaft, R. G., editor: Clinical surgery, the hand, London, 1966, Butterworth and Co., Ltd.
14. Brand, P. W.: Tendon transfers in the forearm. In

Flynn, J. E., editor: Hand surgery, ed. 2, Baltimore, 1975, The Williams & Wilkins Co., pp. 189-200.

15. Brand P. W., Beach R.: Relative tension and potential excursion of muscles in the forearm and hand, J. Hand Surg. **4**:281, 1979.

16. Brooks, A. L., and Jones, D. S.: A new tendon transfer for the paralytic hand. Personal communication, and abstract submitted to American Society for Surgery of the Hand, 1974.

17. Brown, P. W.: Reconstruction of pinch in ulnar intrinsic palsy, Orthop. Clin. North Am. **5**:323, 1974.

18. Bruner, J. M.: Tendon transfer to restore abduction of the index finger using the extensor pollicis brevis, Plast. Reconstr. Surg. **3**:197, 1948.

19. Bunnell, S.: Repair of tendons in the fingers and description of two new instruments, Surg. Gynecol. Obstet. **26**:103, 1918.

20. Bunnell, S.: Repair of tendons in the fingers, Surg. Gynecol. Obstet. **35**:88, 1922.

21. Bunnell, S.: Opposition of the thumb, J. Bone Joint Surg. **20**:269, 1938.

22. Bunnell, S.: Surgery of the intrinsic muscles of the hand other than those producing opposition of the thumb, J. Bone Joint Surg. **24**:1, 1942.

23. Burkhalter, W. E.: Tendon transfers in median nerve palsy, Orthop. Clin. North Am. **5**:271, 1974.

24. Burkhalter, W. E., Christensen, R. C., and Brown, P.: Extensor indicis proprius opponensplasty, J. Bone Joint Surg. **55-A**:725, 1973.

25. Burkhalter, W. E., and Strait, J. L.: Metacarpophalangeal flexor replacement for intrinsic paralysis, J. Bone Joint Surg. **55-A**:1667, 1973.

26. Burman, M. S.: The use of a nylon sheath in the secondary repair of torn finger flexor tendons, Bull. Hosp. Joint Dis. **5**:122, 1944.

27. Camitz, H.: Uber die behandlung der oppositionslahmung, Acta Chir. Scand. **65**:77, 1929.

28. Chaplin, D. M.: The vascular anatomy within normal tendons, divided tendons, free tendon grafts, and pedicle tendon grafts in rabbits, J. Bone Joint Surg. **55-B**:369, 1973.

29. Chong, J. K., Cramer L. M., and Culf, N. K.: Combined two-stage tenoplasty with silicone rods for multiple flexor tendon injuries in "no-man's-land," J. Trauma **12**:104, 1972.

30. Curtis, R. M.: Fundamental principles of tendon transfer, Orthop. Clin. North Am. **5**:231, 1974.

31. Drobnick: Uber die behandlung der kinderlaehmung mit funktionstheilung und funktionsubertragung der muskeln, Dtsch. Ztschr. Chir. **43**:473, 1896.

32. Dums, F.: Über trommeleslähmungen, Dtsch. Militarärzt Ztschr. **25**:145, 1896.

33. Edgerton, M. T., and Brand, P. W.: Restoration of abduction and adduction to the unstable thumb in median and ulnar paralysis, Plast. Reconstr. Surg. **36**:150, 1965.

34. Elftman, H.: Biomechanics of muscle, J. Bone Joint Surg. **48-A**:363, 1966.

35. Fick, A.: Statische berachtung der muskulature des oberschenkels, Z. Rationelle Med. **9**:94, 1850.

36. Flatt, A. E.: The care of the rheumatoid hand, ed. 3, St. Louis, 1974, The C. V. Mosby Co.

37. Freehafer, A. A., Peckham, H., and Keith, M. W.: Determination of muscle-tendon unit properties during tendon transfer, J. Hand Surg. **4**:331, 1979.

38. Fritschi, E. P.: Reconstructive surgery in leprosy, Baltimore, 1971, The Williams & Wilkins Co., pp. 42-88.

39. Furlow, L. T.: The role of tendon tissues in tendon healing, Plast. Reconstr. Surg. **57**:39, 1976.

40. Goenicdtian, S. A.: A new method of canalization tendon sutures with vein grafts, Arch. Surg. **26**:181, 1949.

41. Goldner, J. L.: Deformities of the hand incidental to pathological changes of the extensor and intrinsic muscle mechanisms, J. Bone Joint Surg. **35-A**:115, 1953.

42. Goldner, J. L.: Reconstructive surgery of the hand in cerebral palsy and spastic paralysis resulting from injury to the spinal cord, J. Bone Joint Surg. **37-A**:1141, 1955.

43. Goldner, J. L.: Reconstructive surgery of the upper extremity affected by cerebral palsy or brain or spinal cord trauma. In Current practice in orthopaedic surgery, vol. 3, St. Louis, 1966, The C. V. Mosby Co., pp. 125-138.

44. Goldner, J. L.: Replacement of the function of the paralyzed adductor pollicis with the flexor digitorum sublimis—a ten-year review, J. Bone Joint Surg. **49-A**:583, 1967.

45. Goldner, J. L.: Tendon transfers in rheumatoid arthritis, Orthop. Clin. North Am. **5**:425, 1974.

46. Goldner, J. L.: Upper extremity tendon transfers in cerebral palsy, Orthop. Clin. North Am. **5**:389, 1974.

47. Gonzalez, R. I.: Experimental tendon repair within the flexor tunnels: use of polyethylene tubes for improvement of functional results in the dog, Surgery **26**:181, 1949.

48. Gonzalez, R. I.: Experimental use of teflon in tendon surgery, Plast. Reconstr. Surg. **22**:562, 1958.

49. Green, W. T., and McDermott, L. J.: Operative treatment of cerebral palsy of spastic type, J.A.M.A. **118**:434, 1942.

50. Hanisch, C. M., and Kleiger, B.: Experimental production of tendon sheaths. A preliminary report on the implantation of a flexible plastic in the tissues of rabbits and guinea pigs, Bull. Hosp. Joint Dis. **9**:22, 1948.

51. Henderson, E. D.: Transfer of wrist extensors and brachioradialis to restore opposition of the thumb, J. Bone Joint Surg. **44-A**:513, 1962.

52. Henze, C. W., and Mayer, L.: An experimental study of silk-tendon plastics with particular reference to the prevention of postoperative adhesions, Surg. Gynecol. Obstet. **19**:10, 1914.

53. Hochstrasser, A. E., Broadbert, T. R., and Woolf, R.: Sheath replacement in tendon repair. Experimental study with Ivalon, Rocky Mt. Med. J. **57**:30, 1960.

54. Huber, E.: Hilfsoperation bei medianuslahmung, Dtsch. Z. Chir. **162**:271, 1921.

55. Hunter, J. M., Salem, A. W., Steindel, G. R., and Salisbury, R. E.: The use of gliding artifical tendon implants to form new tendon beds. In Proceedings of the American Society for Surgery of the Hand, J. Bone Joint Surg. **51-A**:790, 1969.

56. Hunter, J. M., and Salisbury, R. E.: Flexor tendon reconstruction in severely damaged hands. A two-stage procedure using a silicone-dacron reinforced gliding prosthesis prior to tendon grafting, J. Bone Joint Surg. **53-A**:829, 1971.

57. Hunter, J. M., and Schneider, L. H.: Staged flexor ten-

don reconstruction: current status. In American Academy of Orthopaedic Surgeons: Symposium on tendon surgery in the hand, St. Louis, 1974, The C. V. Mosby Co., pp. 271-274.

58. Jones, R.: Tendon transplantation in cases of musculospiral injuries not amenable to suture, Am. J. Surg. **35:**333, 1921.

59. Kaplan, E. B.: Functional and surgical anatomy of the hand, ed. 2, Philadelphia, 1965, J. B. Lippincott, Co.

60. Lange, F.: Die sehnenverpflanzung, Ergebr. Chir Orthop. **2:**1, 1911.

61. Lanz, V. T., and Wachsmuth, W.: Praktische Anatomie erster band. Driter Teil. Arm., Berlin, 1935, Julius Springer, pp. 154-243.

62. Leffert, R. D., and Meister, M.: Patterns of neuromuscular activity following tendon transfer in the upper limb: a preliminary study, J. Bone Joint Surg. **3:**181, 1976.

63. Lipscomb, P. R., Elkins, E. C., and Henderson, E. D.: Tendon transfers to restore function of hands in tetraplegia, especially after fracture-dislocation of the sixth cervical vertebra on the seventh, J. Bone Joint Surg. **40-A:**1071, 1958.

64. Littler, J. W.: Tendon transfer and arthrodesis in combined median and ulnar nerve paralysis, J. Bone Joint Surg. **31-A:**225, 1949.

65. Littler, J. W., and Cooley, S. G. S.: Opposition of the thumb and its restoration by abductor digiti quinti transfer, J. Bone Joint Surg. **45-A:**1389, 1963.

66. Littler, J. W., and Li, C. S.: Primary restoration of thumb opposition with median nerve decompression, Plast. Reconstr. Surg. **39:**74, 1967.

67. Lundborg, G., Myrhage, R., and Rydevik, B.: The vascularization of human flexor tendons within the digital synovial sheath region—structural and functional aspects, J. Hand Surg. **2:**417, 1977.

68. Makin, M.: Translocation of the flexor pollicis longus tendon to restore opposition, J. Bone Joint Surg. **49-B:**458, 1967.

69. Mannerfelt, L., and Norman, O.: Attrition ruptures of flexor tendons in rheumatoid arthritis caused by bony spurs in the carpal tunnel, J. Bone Joint Surg. **51-B:**270, 1969.

70. Manske, P. R., Lesker, P. A., and Bridwell, K.: Experimental studies on the initial nutrition of flexor tendon grafts, J. Hand Surg. **4:**282, 1979.

71. Mayer, L.: The physiological method of tendon transplantation. I. Historical: anatomy and physiology of tendons, Surg. Gynecol. Obstet. **22:**182, 1916.

72. Mayer, L.: The physiological method of tendon transplantation. II. Operative technique, Surg. Gynecol. Obstet. **22:**298, 1916.

73. Mayer, L.: The physiological method of tendon transplantation. III. Experimental and clinical experiences, Surg. Gynecol. Obstet. **22:**422, 1916.

74. Mayer, L.: The physiological method of tendon transplantation, Surg. Gynecol. Obstet. **33:**528, 1921.

75. Mayer, L., and Ransohoff, N.: Reconstruction of the digital tendon sheath, J. Bone Surg. **18:**607, 1936.

76. McDowell, C. L.: Tendon healing. An experimental model in the dog, J. Hand Surg. **2:**122, 1977.

77. Milgram, J. E.: Tendon transplantation of biceps and tri-

ceps to paralyzed fingers through artifically erected tendon sheaths, Bull. Hosp. Joint Dis. **15:**45, 1954.

78. Milgram, J. E.: Transplantation of tendons through performed gliding channels, Bull. Hosp. Joint Dis. **21:**250, 1960.

79. Millender, L. H., and Nalebuff, E. A., et al.: Dorsal tenosynovectomy and tendon transfer in the rheumatoid hand, J. Bone Joint Surg. **56-A:**601, 1974.

80. Nalebuff, E. A.: The recognition and treatment of tendon ruptures in the rheumatoid hand. In American Academy of Orthopaedic Surgeons: Symposium on tendon surgery in the hand, St. Louis, 1974, The C. V. Mosby Co., pp. 255-270.

81. Nalebuff, E. A., and Patel, M. R.: Flexor digitorum sublimis transfer for multiple extensor tendon ruptures in rheumatoid arthritis, Plast. Reconstr. Surg. **52:**530, 1973.

82. Neviaser, R. J., Wilson, J. N., and Gardner, M. M.: Abductor pollicis longus transfer for replacement of first dorsal interosseous, J. Hand Surg. **5:**53, 1980.

83. Ney, K. W.: A tendon transplant for intrinsic hand muscle paralysis, Surg. Gynecol. Obstet. **33:**342, 1921.

84. Nichols, H. M.: Discussion of tendon repair with clinical and experimental data on the use of gelatin sponge, Ann. Surg. **129:**223, 1949.

85. Nicoladoni, K.: Uber sehnentransplantation. Nersamml. Deutsch Naturforsch. Artzle in Salsburg, Vol. 54, 1880.

86. Nicoladoni, K.: Nachtrag zur pes calcaneus und zur transplantation der peronealsehnen, Arch. Klin. Chir. **27:**660, 1882.

87. Ochiai, N., Matsui, T., Miyaji, N., Merklin, R. J., and Hunter, J. M.: Vascular anatomy of flexor tendons. I. Vascular system and blood supply of the profundus tendon in the digital sheath, J. Hand Surg. **4:**321, 1979.

88. Omer, G. E., Jr.: Determination of physiological length of a reconstructed muscle tendon unit through muscle stimulation, J. Bone Joint Surg. **47-A:**304, 1965.

89. Omer, G. E., Jr.: Tendon transfers in combined nerve injury, Orthop. Clin. North Am. **5:**377, 1974.

90. Paneva-Holevich, E.: Two-stage tenoplasty in injury of the flexor tendons of the hand, J. Bone Joint Surg. **51-A:**21, 1969.

91. Peacock, E. E., Jr.: A study of the circulation in normal tendons and healing graft, Ann. Surg. **149:**415, 1959.

92. Phalen, G. S., and Miller, R. C.: The transfer of wrist extensor muscles to restore or reinforce flexion power of the fingers and opposition of the thumb, J. Bone Joint Surg. **29:**993, 1947.

93. Ramselaar, J. M.: Tendon transfer to restore opposition of the thumb, Leiden, Holland, 1970, H. E. Stenfert Kroese.

94. Riordan, D. C.: Surgery of the paralytic hand. In American Academy of Orthopaedic Surgeons: Instructional course lectures, vol. 16, St. Louis, 1959, The C. V. Mosby Co., pp. 79-90.

95. Riordan, D. C.: Tendon transfers for nerve paralysis of the hand and wrist. In Current practice in orthopaedic surgery, vol. 2, St. Louis, 1964,The C. V. Mosby Co., pp. 17-40.

96. Salisbury, R. E., Levine N. S., McKeel, D. W., Pruitt, B. A., and Wade, C. W. R.: Tendon sheath reconstruction with artificial implants: a study of ultrastructure. In

American Academy of Orthopaedic Surgeons: Symposium on tendon surgery in the hand, St. Louis, 1965, The C. V. Mosby Co., pp. 59-65.

97. Seddon, H. T.: Surgical disorders of the peripheral nerves, Baltimore, 1972, The Williams & Wilkins Co., pp. 28-31, and 171-172.

98. Smith, R. J.: Balance and kinetics of the fingers under normal and pathological conditions, Clin. Orthop. **104:**92, 1974.

99. Smith, R. J.: Intrinsic muscles of the fingers: function, dysfunction, and surgical reconstruction. In American Academy of Orthopaedic Surgeons: Instructional course lectures, vol. 24, St. Louis, 1975, The C. V. Mosby Co., pp. 200-220.

100. Smith, R. J.: Surgical treatment of the clawhand. In American Academy of Orthopaedic Surgeons: Symposium on tendon surgery in the hand, St. Louis, 1975, The C. V. Mosby Co., pp. 181-203.

101. Smith, R. J., and Broudy, A. S.: Advances in surgery of the rheumatoid hand. In Current practice in orthopaedic surgery, vol. 7, St. Louis, 1977, The C. V. Mosby Co., pp. 1-35.

102. Steindler, A.: Nutrition and vitality of the tendon in tendon transplantation, Am. J. Orthop. Surg. **16:**63, 1918.

103. Steindler, A.: Orthopaedic operations on the hand, J.A.M.A. **71:**1288, 1918.

104. Steindler, A.: Orthopaedic operations: indications, technique, and end results, Springfield, Ill., 1940, Charles C. Thomas, Publisher.

105. Steindler, A.: Transplantation of tendons at the elbow. In American Academy of Orthopaedic Surgeons: Instructional course lectures. Ann Arbor, Mich., 1944, J. W. Edwards, pp. 276-283.

106. Steindler, A.: The reconstruction of upper extremity in spinal and cerebral paralysis. In American Academy of Orthopaedic Surgeons: Instructional course lectures, vol. 6, Ann Arbor, Mich. 1949, J. W. Edwards, pp. 120-133.

107. Steindler, A.: Reconstruction of the poliomyelitic upper extremity, Bull. Hosp. Joint Dis. **15:**21, 1954.

108. Steindler, A.: Kinesiology of the human body, Springfield, Ill., 1955, Charles C Thomas, Publisher.

109. Stiles, H. J., and Forrester-Brown, M. F.: Treatment of injuries of the peripheral spinal nerves, London, 1922, H. Frowde, p. 166.

110. Stoffel, A.: Verhandl. d. deutsch. orthop. Gesellsch., 1913 and 1914.

111. Straub, L. R.: The rheumatoid hand, Clin. Orthop. **15:**127, 1959.

112. Straub, L. R., and Wilson, E. H., Jr.: Spontaneous rupture of extensor tendons in the hand associated with rheumatoid arthritis, J. Bone Joint Surg., **38-A:**1208, 1956.

113. Thatcher, H.: Use of stainless steel rods to canalize flexor tendon sheaths, South. Med. J. **32:**13, 1939.

114. Thompson, T. C.: A modified operation for opponens paralysis, J. Bone Joint Surg. **24:**632, 1942.

115. Tubiana, R.: Anatomic and physiologic basis for the surgical treatment of paralysis of the hand, J. Bone Joint Surg. **51-A:**643, 1969.

116. Weber, W., and Weber E.: Machanik der menschlichen Gehwerkzeuge, Gottingen, 1836, Dieterich.

117. Wheeldon, T.: The use of cellophane as a permanent tendon sheath, J. Bone Joint Surg. **21:**393, 1939.

118. Williams, H. W. G.: The leprosy thumb, Br. J. Plast. Surg. **19:**136, 1966.

119. Urbaniack, J. R., Bright, D. S., Gill, L. H., and Goldner, J. L.: Vascularization and the gliding mechanism of free flexor tendon grafts inserted by the silicone-rod method, J. Bone Joint Surg. **56-A:**473, 1974.

120. Vaughan-Jackson, O. J.: Rupture of extensor tendons by attrition at the inferior radio-ulnar joint. Report of two cases, J. Bone Joint Surg. **30-B:**528, 1948.

121. Vaughan-Jackson, O. J.: Attrition ruptures of tendons in the rheumatoid hand, J. Bone Joint Surg. **40-A:**1431, 1958.

122. Vaughan-Jackson, O. J.: Tendon rupture in the rheumatoid hand, J. Bone Joint Surg. **41-B:**629, 1959.

123. Vulpius: Zeitschrift für Orth. Chir., **12:**1, 1904.

124. Vulpius and Stoffel: Die behandlung der spinalen kinderlaehmung. As cited in Mayer, L.: The physiological method of tendon transplantation. I. Historical: anatomy and physiology of tendons, Surg. Gynecol. Obstet. **22:**182, 1916.

125. Zancolli, E.: Tendon transfers after ischemic contracture of the forearm, Am. J. Surg. **109:**356, 1965.

126. Zancolli, E.: Structural and dynamic bases of hand surgery, Philadelphia, 1968, J. B. Lippincott Co.

127. Zancolli, E.: Correccion de la "garra" digital por paralisis intrinseca; la operacion del "lazo," Acta. Orthop. Latinoamericana **1:**65, 1974.

128. Zweig, J., Rosenthal, S., and Burns, H.: Transfer of the extensor digiti quinti to restore pinch in ulnar palsy of the hand, J. Bone Joint Surg. **54-A:**51, 1972.

Index